Learn Medical Spanish in 100 Days

Spanish Words & Phrases for Healthcare Professionals to Become Fluent Faster

TOURI

ISBN: 9781953149084

DISCLAIMER

Practitioners should not rely on the content of this book to evaluate, diagnose or treat medical conditions. The information in this book is meant only to serve as a tool for health care providers who want to improve their ability to communicate with their Spanish-speaking patients; it does not replace the services of a trained medical interpreter (which may be required by law).

WANT THE AUDIOBOOK FOR FREE?

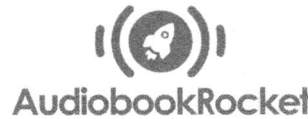

We have a **limited** amount of **free** promotional codes for this audiobook.

Here's how it works:

1. **Visit the link below** to see the listing on AudiobookRocket
2. Request a free promo code from us
3. In **30 days** leave an honest, unbiased review on the audiobook.
4. Confirm & notify us on AudiobookRocket that you left a review.
5. Request and enjoy additional audiobooks from other publishers on the site.

https://audiobookrocket.com/audiobooks/11

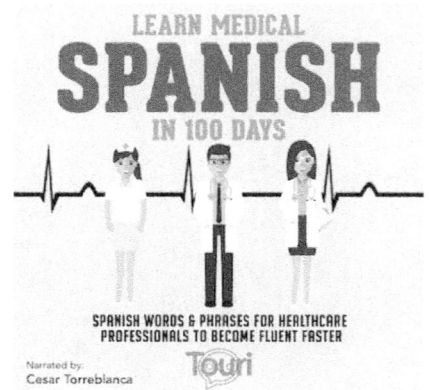

IF YOU ENJOY THE FREE AUDIOBOOK,

PLEASE HELP US OUT AND **LEAVE A REVIEW**

Table of Contents

INTRODUCTION 1

RESOURCES 2

FREE SPANISH VIDEO COURSE 5

QUICK REFERENCE OF COMMON WORDS & PHRASES 6

DAY 1 16

DAY 2 18

DAY 3 20

DAY 4 22

DAY 5 25

DAY 6 28

DAY 7 30

DAY 8 32

DAY 9 34

DAY 10 36

DAY 11 39

DAY 12 42

DAY 13 45

DAY 14 48

DAY 15 51

DAY 16 54

DAY 17 57

DAY 18 60

DAY 19 63

DAY 20 66

DAY 21 69

DAY 22	72
DAY 23	75
DAY 24	78
DAY 25	81
DAY 26	84
DAY 27	87
DAY 28	90
DAY 29	93
DAY 30	96
DAY 31	99
DAY 32	102
DAY 33	105
DAY 34	107
DAY 35	109
DAY 36	112
DAY 37	114
DAY 38	116
DAY 39	118
DAY 40	120
DAY 41	123
DAY 42	125
DAY 43	127
DAY 44	129
DAY 45	131
DAY 46	134
DAY 47	136
DAY 48	138

DAY 49   140

DAY 50   143

DAY 51   145

DAY 52   147

DAY 53   149

DAY 54   151

DAY 55   153

DAY 56   155

DAY 57   157

DAY 58   159

DAY 59   161

DAY 60   163

DAY 61   165

DAY 62   167

DAY 63   169

DAY 64   171

DAY 65   173

DAY 66   175

DAY 67   177

DAY 68   179

DAY 69   181

DAY 70   183

DAY 71   185

DAY 72   187

DAY 73   189

DAY 74   191

DAY 75   193

DAY 76   195

DAY 77   197

DAY 78   199

DAY 79   201

DAY 80   203

DAY 81   205

DAY 82   207

DAY 83   209

DAY 84   211

DAY 85   213

DAY 86   215

DAY 87   217

DAY 88   219

DAY 89   221

DAY 90   223

DAY 91   225

DAY 92   227

DAY 93   229

DAY 94   231

DAY 95   233

DAY 96   235

DAY 97   237

DAY 98   239

DAY 99   241

DAY 100   243

DIALOGUES   245

DOLOR ABDOMINAL – ABDOMINAL PAIN   245

DOLOR DE LA ESPALDA – BACK PAIN   247

DOLOR DE PECHO – CHEST PAIN   249

ESTREÑIMIENTO – CONSTIPATION   251

DEPRESIÓN – DEPRESSION   253

DIARREA – DIARRHEA   255

MAREO – DIZZINESS   257

DOLOR DE OIDOS – EARACHE   259

DOLOR DE CABEZA – HEADACHE   261

INSOMNIO – INSOMNIA   263

DOLOR DE RODILLAS – KNEE PAIN   265

DOLOR DE CUELLO – NECK PAIN   267

DOLOR DE OJOS / OJOS ROJOS – RED / PAINFUL EYE   269

FALTA DE ALIENTO – SHORTNESS OF BREATH   271

DOLOR DE HOMBROS – SHOULDER PAIN   273

DOLOR DE LA GARGANTA – SORE THROAT   275

INFECCIÓN RESPIRATORIA SUPERIOR – UPPER RESPIRATORY INFECTION   277

INFECCIÓN DEL APARATO URINARIO – URINARY TRACT INFECTION   279

ABOUT THE AUTHOR   282

OTHER BOOKS BY TOURI   283

FREE AUDIOBOOKS   287

INTRODUCTION

We want to thank you and congratulate you for purchasing *"Learn Medical Spanish in 100 Days"*.

This book contains a daily list of 10 helpful vocabulary words and phrases in English and Spanish to breakdown the communication barriers. In addition, there are helpful conversational dialogues between a doctor and patient with common scenarios in which you may find yourself.

By using this book as a guide, learning just one real world phrase a day will dramatically improve your Spanish comprehension and verbal capabilities ultimately allowing you to focus on providing world-class care in the Spanish language.

Thanks again for purchasing this book, we hope you enjoy it!

Now get out there and speak eloquently!

RESOURCES

TOURI.CO

One of the best ways to learn this material is through repetition, memorization and conversation. If you'd like to practice your newly learned vocabulary, Touri offers live fun and immersive 1-on-1 online language lessons with native instructors at nearly anytime of the day. For more information go to Touri.co now.

FACEBOOK GROUP
Learn Spanish - Touri Language Learning
Learn French - Touri Language Learning

YOUTUBE
Touri Language Learning Channel

ANDROID APP
Learn Spanish App for Beginners

BOOKS

GERMAN

Conversational German Dialogues: 50 German Conversations and Short Stories

German Short Stories (Volume 1): 10 Exciting Short Stories to Easily Learn German & Improve Your Vocabulary

ITALIAN

Conversational Italian Dialogues: 50 Italian Conversations and Short Stories

Italian Short Stories (Volume 1): 10 Exciting Short Stories to Easily Learn Italian & Improve Your Vocabulary

SPANISH

Conversational Spanish Dialogues: 50 Spanish Conversations and Short Stories

Spanish Short Stories (Volume 1): 10 Exciting Short Stories to Easily Learn Spanish & Improve Your Vocabulary

Spanish Short Stories (Volume 2): 10 Exciting Short Stories to Easily Learn Spanish & Improve Your Vocabulary

Intermediate Spanish Short Stories (Volume 1): 10 Amazing Short Tales to Learn Spanish & Quickly Grow Your Vocabulary the Fun Way!

Intermediate Spanish Short Stories (Volume 2): 10 Amazing Short Tales to Learn Spanish & Quickly Grow Your Vocabulary the Fun Way!

100 Days of Real World Spanish: Useful Words & Phrases for All Levels to Help You Become Fluent Faster

Learn Medical Spanish in 100 Days: Spanish Words & Phrases for Healthcare Professionals to Become Fluent Faster

FRENCH

Conversational French Dialogues: 50 French Conversations and Short Stories

French Short Stories for Beginners (Volume 1): 10 Exciting Short Stories to Easily Learn French & Improve Your Vocabulary

French Short Stories for Beginners (Volume 2): 10 Exciting Short Stories to Easily Learn French & Improve Your Vocabulary

Intermediate French Short Stories (Volume 1): 10 Amazing Short Tales to Learn French & Quickly Grow Your Vocabulary the Fun Way!

PORTUGUESE

Conversational Portuguese Dialogues: 50 Portuguese Conversations and Short Stories

ARABIC

Conversational Arabic Dialogues: 50 Arabic Conversations and Short Stories

RUSSIAN

Conversational Russian Dialogues: 50 Russian Conversations and Short Stories

CHINESE

Conversational Chinese Dialogues: 50 Chinese Conversations and Short Stories

FREE SPANISH VIDEO COURSE

200+ words and phrases in audio
you can start using today!
Get it while it's available

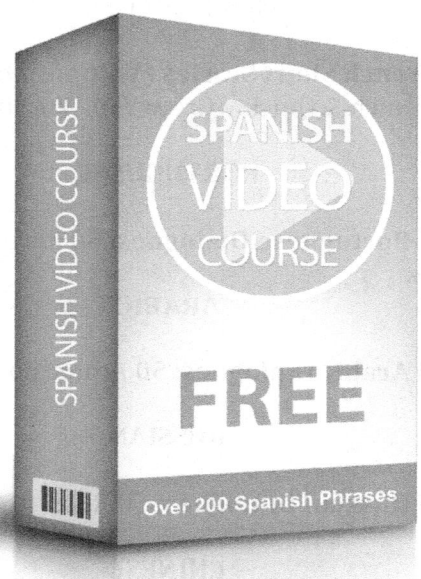

https://bit.ly/Medical-Spanish-Free-Video-Course

QUICK REFERENCE OF COMMON WORDS & PHRASES

GREETINGS AND FAREWELLS

Good morning	Buenos días
Good afternoon	Buenas tardes
Good night	Buenas noches
Hi	Hola
Goodbye	Hasta luego
Sir	Señor
Mrs.	Señora
Miss	Señorita

SOCIAL PLEASANTRIES AND COURTESY

Please	Por favor
Thank you	Gracias
Excuse me	Perdón
You're welcome	De nada
How are you feeling today?	¿Cómo se siente hoy?
Are you feeling better?	¿Se siente mejor?
Have a good day	Que tenga un buen día
I'm sorry	Lo siento

INTRODUCTIONS

I'm the nurse	Soy la enfermera
I'll be taking care of you today	Yo voy a cuidar de usted hoy
My name is_____.	Mi nombre es _____.
What's your name?	¿Cuál es su nombre?
Nice to meet you	Mucho gusto.
Please sit down	Por favor, siéntese
This is the nurse's aide	Este es el auxiliar de enfermería
This is the doctor	Este es el doctor
Do you need an interpreter?	¿Necesita un intérprete?

STRATEGIES FOR BETTER COMMUNICATIONS

Do you speak English?	¿Habla Inglés?
I don't speak Spanish	Yo no hablo español
I only speak a little Spanish	Yo sólo hablo un poco de español
Do you understand?	¿Me entiende?
I don't understand	No entiendo
Repeat that, please	Repita eso, por favor
Please, only answer "yes" or "no"	Por favor, sólo responda sí o no
Speak very slowly, please	Por favor, hable despacio

TALKING ABOUT FAMILY

Do you have children?	¿Tiene hijos?
What's your relation to Mr. Morgan?	¿Cuál es su relación con el Sr. Morgan?
Is he your son?	¿Él es su hijo?
Is she your daughter?	¿Ella es su hija?
Are you her husband?	¿Es usted el esposo de ella?
Are you his wife?	¿Es usted la esposa de él?
Is he your brother?	¿Él es su hermano?
Is she your sister?	¿Ella es su hermana?

PATIENT ORIENTATION

This is your room	Este es su cuarto
This is your bed	Esta es su cama
This button will raise and lower the bed	Este botón sube y baja la cama
Please keep the side rails up	Por favor, tenga las barandas arriba
Push this button if you need help	Pulse este botón si necesita ayuda
The telephone is here	El teléfono está aquí
Here's the control for the television	Aquí está el control de la televisión
The bathroom is here	El baño está aquí

NUMBERS

Zero	Cero
One	Uno
Two	Dos
Three	Tres
Four	Cuatro
Five	Cinco
Six	Seis
Seven	Siete
Eight	Ocho
Nine	Nueve
Ten	Dez
Twenty	Veinte
Thirty	Treinta
Forty	Cuarenta
Fifty	Cincuenta
Sixty	Sesenta
Seventy	Setenta
Eighty	Ochenta
Ninety	Noventa
Hundred	Cien

TAKING VITALS

I'm going to take your blood pressure	Voy a tomar la presión arterial
I'm going to take your temperature	Voy a tomar la temperatura
I'm going to take your pulse	Voy a tomar el pulso
I'm going to listen to your lungs	Voy a escuchar sus pulmones
Breathe deeply, please	Respire profundamente, por favor
I'm going to listen to your heart	Voy a escuchar a su corazón
Everything is normal	Todo es normal

AMBULATION

I'm going to help you get into the chair	Voy a ayudarlo a sentarse en la silla
Hold on to me	Aférrese a mí
I want you to stand up	Quiero que usted se levante
Hold the walker	Sostenga el andador
Let's walk down the hallway	Vamos a caminar por el pasillo
I won't let you fall	Yo no lo voy a dejar caer
Don't get out of bed without help	No salga de la cama sin ayuda
You can't walk by yourself	No puede caminar por sí mismo

POSITIONING

Turn on your right side	Gire a tu derecha
Turn on your left side	Gire a tu izquierda
Turn onto your back	Gire en tu espalda
Sit up	Siéntese
Sit on the side of the bed	Siéntese al lado de la cama
Stand up, please	Levántese, por favor

BASIC COMMANDS

Breathe in	Inhale
Breathe out	Exhale
Cough, please	Tosa, por favor
Take this medicine	Tome este medicamento
Listen to me	Escúchame
Wake up	Despiértese
Lie down	Acuéstese
Be careful	Tenga cuidado
Swallow, please	Trague, por favor
Open your mouth	Abra la boca
Please, don't move	No se mueva, por favor
Pay attention	Preste atención

MEDICATIONS

Are you allergic to anything?	¿Es usted alérgico a algo?
Are you currently taking any medications?	¿Toma alguna medicación?
Take this pill	Tome esta pastilla
Take one pill at a time	Tome una pastilla a la vez
This is for the pain	Esto es para el dolor
You need an antibiotic	Usted necesita un antibiótico
I'm going to give you a shot	Voy a darle un inyección
This is going to hurt a little	Esto va a doler un poco

PATIENT COMFORT

Are you having trouble breathing?	¿Está teniendo problemas para respirar?
Did you sleep okay?	¿Ha dormido bien?
Are you cold?	¿Tiene frío?
Are you hot?	¿Tiene calor?
Do you need another blanket?	¿Necesita otra cobija?
Would you like another pillow?	¿Quiere otra almohada?
Are you in pain?	¿Tiene dolor?
Where does it hurt?	¿Dónde le duele?
Touch the spot where it hurts.	Toque donde tiene dolor.

ASSESSING PATIENT ORIENTATION

Do you know where you are?	¿Sabe usted dónde se encuentra?
Do you know why you are here?	¿Sabe usted por qué está aquí?
What day is it?	¿Qué día es hoy?
What month is it?	¿Qué mes es?
Do you know who I am?	¿Sabe usted quién soy yo?

ASSESSING PATIENT COMFORT

Are you hot?	¿Tiene calor?
Are you cold?	¿Tiene frío?
Do you feel OK?	¿Se siente bien?
Do you feel sick?	¿Se siente enfermo?
Are you feeling better?	¿Se siente mejor?

CLEANSING

Did you have a bowel movement?	¿Ha tenido un movimiento estomacal?
I'm going to clean you.	Voy a asearlo.
I'm going to change your diaper.	Voy a cambiar su pañal.
I'm going to change the sheets.	Voy a cambiar las sábanas.
I'm going to bathe you.	Voy a bañarlo.
Can you raise your arms?	¿Puede levantar los brazos?

13

FOOD AND DRINK

Are you hungry?	¿Tiene hambre?
Are you thirsty?	¿Tiene sed?
Do you have problems chewing?	¿Tiene problemas para masticar?
Do you have problems swallowing?	¿Tiene problemas para tragar?
I'm going to help you eat.	Voy a ayudarlo a comer.
Here's your breakfast.	Aquí está su desayuno.
Here's your lunch.	Aquí está su almuerzo.
Here's your dinner.	Aquí está su cena.

DRESSING

Put on your shirt.	Póngase la camisa.
Put on your socks.	Póngase las medias.
Put on your pants.	Póngase los pantalones.
Remove your shirt.	Quítese la camisa.
Remove your socks.	Quítese las medias.
Remove your pants.	Quítese los pantalones.

POSITIVITY & GOOD CHEER

You'll be going home soon!	Usted se va para su casa pronto!
You have a wonderful family!	Usted tiene una familia maravillosa!
You're doing great!	Que está haciendo muy bien!
Sleep well!	Duerma bien!

14

You're looking much better!	Se le ve mucho mejor!
Are you feeling worse?	¿Se siente peor?

BATHROOM

Do you need to use the bathroom?	¿Necesita usar el baño?
Here's the bathroom.	Aquí está el baño.
I'll help you bathe.	Lo voy a ayudar a bañarse.
Try to urinate.	Trate de orinar.

EATING

Pick up your fork.	Recoja tu tenedor.
Put down your spoon.	Deje tu cuchara.
Scoop up some food.	Recoja algo de comida.
Chew well and then swallow.	Mastique bien antes de tragar.
Pick up your cup.	Recoja tu taza.
Take a drink.	Tome un sorbo.
Not too much.	No mucho.
Wipe your mouth.	Límpiese la boca.

DAY 1

Human Body - Part 1

1. Tobillo - (Toh-bee-yoh)
Translation: Ankle
English: He broke his ankle from falling off his bike.
Spanish: Se rompió el tobillo al caer de la bicicleta.

2. Brazo - (Brah-zoh)
Translation: Arm
English: Extend your arms
Spanish: extienda/estire sus brazos

3. Axila, "sobaco" - (ax-ee-luh, so-bah-co)
Translation: Armpit
English: In the old days, women did not shave their armpits
Spanish: Antiguamente las mujeres no se depilaban las axilas.

4. Espalda - (Es-pahl-duh)
Translation: Back
English: My back hurts
Spanish: Me duele la espalda

5. Seno - (Seh-noh)
Translation: Breast
English: My aunt had a cyst removed from her right breast.
Spanish: A mi tía le extirparon un quiste de su seno derecho.

6. Pecho - (Pay-cho)

Translation: Chest

English: The doctor asked him to take off his shirt to listen to his chest.

Spanish: El doctor le pidió que se quitara la camisa para auscultarle el pecho.

7. Mejilla - (Meh-hee-yuh)

Translation: Cheek

English: They slapped him on the cheek.

Spanish: Le dieron una bofetada en la mejilla.

8. T mpano del o do - (Teem-pah-noh del oh-EE-doh)

Translation: Eardrum

English: The eardrum separates the middle ear from the outer ear.

Spanish: El tímpano separa el oído medio del externo.

9. Codo - (Coh-doh)

Translation: Elbow

English: Jaime can't bend his right arm because he's broken his elbow.

Spanish: Jaime no puede doblar el brazo derecho porque se rompió el codo.

10. Ojo - (Oh-hoe)

Translation: Eye

English: He doesn't see well through his right eye.

Spanish: No ve bien por el ojo derecho.

DAY 2

HUMAN BODY - PART 2

11. Barbilla, ment n - (Bar-bee-yah)
Translation: Chin
English: That handsome man has a cleft chin.
Spanish: Es un hombre apuesto de barbilla partida.

12. Ano - (Ah-no)
Translation: Anus
English: He had a fistula on the anus and had to be operated on.
Spanish: Tuvieron que operarlo de una fístula en el ano.

13. Ceja - (Say-ha)
Translation: Eyebrow
English: He had bright blue eyes that contrasted with his dark eyebrows.
Spanish: Él tenía ojos azules brillantes que contrastaban con sus cejas oscuras.

14. Pesta as - (Pes-tahn-yahs)
Translation: Eyelashes
English: I burned my eyelashes when I got too close to the candle.
Spanish: Se me quemaron las pestañas al acercarme demasiado a la vela.

15. Dedo - (Day-doh)
Translation: Finger/toes
English: I cut my finger making dinner.
Spanish: Me corté el dedo haciendo la cena.

16. Pie - (Pee-ay)

Translation: Foot

English: I sprained my right foot playing soccer.

Spanish: Me hice un esguince en el pie derecho mientras jugaba fútbol.

17. Frente - (Fren-tay)

Translation: Forehead

English: He's got a noticeable wrinkle on his forehead.

Spanish: Tiene una profunda arruga en la frente.

18. Mano - (Mah-no)

Translation: Hand

English: I took the old man by the hand to help him cross the street.

Spanish: Tomé al anciano de la mano para ayudarlo a cruzar la calle.

19. Cabeza - (Kah-bay-sah)

Translation: Head

English: I didn't look where I was going and I hit my head.

Spanish: No miré por dónde andaba y me di un golpe en la cabeza.

20. Cadera - (Kah-dare-uh)

Translation: Hip

English: Philip rolled down the stairs and broke his hip. He won't be able to walk for a while.

Spanish: Felipe se rodó por las escaleras y se fracturó la cadera, no podrá caminar por un tiempo.

DAY 3

HUMAN BODY - PART 3

21. Conducto/canal auditivo - (Cone-dook-toe awe-dee-tee-voh)
Translation: Ear canal
English: Sound passes through the ear canal.
Spanish: El sonido pasa por el conducto auditivo.

22. P rpado - (PAR-pa-doh)
Translation: Eyelid
English: She pretended to be asleep, but her eyelids were half-open.
Spanish: Fingía estar dormida, pero tenía los párpados entreabiertos.

23. Tal n - (Tah-lone)
Translation: Heel
English: I can't walk because I injured my heel while playing basketball.
Spanish: No puedo caminar porque me lastimé el talón mientras jugaba al baloncesto.

24. Mand bula - (Man-dee-boo-lah)
Translation: Jaw/mandible
English: Her jaw/mandible was dislocated in a car accident.
Spanish: Se dislocó la mandíbula en un accidente de tránsito.

25. Rodilla - (Roh-dee-ya)
Translation: Knee
English: The basketball player injured his knee.
Spanish: El jugador de baloncesto se lesionó la rodilla.

26. Pierna - (Pee-air-nuh)

Translation: Leg

English: I injured my leg playing football.

Spanish: Me lesioné la pierna jugando fútbol.

27. Labios - (Lah-bee-yohs)

Translation: Lips

English: My swollen lips wouldn't let a single sound through.

Spanish: Mis labios hinchados no dejaron pasar ningún sonido.

28. Boca - (Bow-kah)

Translation: Mouth

English: I opened my mouth so the dentist could examine my teeth.

Spanish: Abrí la boca para que el dentista pudiera examinar los dientes.

29. Espinilla - (Es-pee-nee-yah)

Translation: Shin

English: I hit my shin on the table leg.

Spanish: Me di un golpe en la espinilla con la pata de la mesa.

30. Mu eca - (Moon-yay-kah)

Translation: Wrist

English: I hurt my wrist when I fell down.

Spanish: Me hice daño en la muñeca cuando me caí.

DAY 4

CIRCULATORY SYSTEM - SISTEMA CIRCULATORIO

31. Aorta - (Ay-or-tah)
Translation: Aorta
English: Oxygenated blood exits the heart through the aorta, bringing oxygen to the rest of the body.
Spanish: La sangre oxigenada sale del corazón por la aorta, llevando oxígeno al resto del cuerpo.

32. Arteria - (Ar-ter-EE-uh)
Translation: Artery
English: The cardiologist told me I had a blocked artery.
Spanish: El cardiólogo me dijo que tenía una arteria obstruida.

33. Coraz n - (Cor-uh-zohn)
Translation: Heart
English: I can hear my heart beating.
Spanish: Puedo oír el latido de mi corazón.

34. Vena yugular - (Vay-nuh yag-oo-lar)
Translation: Jugular vein
English: The jugular vein refers to each of the two that are found in the neck.
Spanish: Se llama vena yugular cada una de las dos que se encuentran en el cuello.

35. Bazo - (Bah-zoh)
Translation: Spleen
English: The doctor palpated the area of the spleen and confirmed it had swollen up due to the infection.
Spanish: El médico palpó la zona del bazo y comprobó que se había inflamado debido a la infección.

36. Vena - (Vay-nuh)
Translation: Vein
English: The nurse had a hard time finding the vein in my arm to draw blood.
Spanish: A la enfermera se le hizo difícil encontrar la vena en mi brazo para sacar sangre.

DIGESTIVE SYSTEM - SISTEMA DIGESTIVO

37. Apéndice - (Ah-PEN-dee-say)
Translation: Appendix
English: My sister had an inflamed appendix, but she didn't have to have it removed.
Spanish: Mi hermana tenía el apéndice inflamado, pero no se lo operaron.

38. Esófago, "boca del estómago" - (Es-OFF-ago, Bow-kah del es-TOH-mah-go)
Translation: Esophagus
English: The doctors were able to reconstruct the patient's damaged esophagus.
Spanish: Los médicos pudieron reconstruir el esófago dañado del paciente.

39. Vesícula biliar - (Ves-EE-coo-lah bee-lee-ar)
Translation: Gallbladder
English: The doctor said that he's going to take an ultrasound of my gallbladder.
Spanish: El médico dijo que va a sacar un ultrasonido de la vesícula biliar.

40. Intestinos, "tripas" - (In-tes-TEE-nohs, tree-pahs)
Translation: Intestines
English: The large intestine is wider and shorter than the small intestine.
Spanish: El intestino grueso es más ancho y más corto que el intestino delgado.

41. H gado - (EE-gah-doh)
Translation: Liver
English: My grandfather has to take medication because he has problems with his liver.
Spanish: Mi abuelo tiene que tomar medicamentos porque tiene problemas con el hígado.

42. P ncreas - (PAN-cree-uhs)
Translation: Pancreas
English: The pancreas secretes several enzymes essential for the digestion of protein.
Spanish: El páncreas segrega varias enzimas esenciales para la digestión de las proteínas.

43. Est mago - (Es-TOH-mah-go)
Translation: Stomach
English: She was complaining of an upset stomach after eating fifteen tacos.
Spanish: Se quejó de un malestar del estomago después de comer quince tacos.

44. Recto - (Reck-toh)
Translation: Rectum
English: The tumor was discovered after an inspection of the colon, rectum, and anus.
Spanish: El tumor fue descubierto gracias a una inspección de colon, recto y ano.

DAY 5

SKELETAL SYSTEM - SISTEMA OSEO

45. Hueso - (way-soh)
Translation: Bone
English: The human skeleton is composed of 206 bones.
Spanish: El esqueleto humano se compone de 206 huesos.

46. Clav cula - (clah-VEE-coo-lah)
Translation: Clavicle
English: Ana's so thin that her collarbone really sticks out.
Spanish: Ana está tan delgada que tiene la clavícula muy marcada.

47. F mur - (FEH-mur)
Translation: Femur
English: The anthropologists found a Neanderthal's femur at the dig site.
Spanish: Los antropólogos encontraron un fémur de un neanderthal en el sitio de excavación.

48. Pelvis - (pel-vis)
Translation: Pelvis
English: Sexually transmitted infections also frequently cause pelvic inflammatory disease, which often produces infertility.
Spanish: Las infecciones de transmisión sexual también están vinculadas con frecuencia a la enfermedad inflamatoria de la pelvis, que a menudo es causa de esterilidad.

49. Costilla - (kohs-stee-yah)

Translation: Rib

English: The doctor said the car crash broke one of my ribs.

Spanish: El médico dijo que me había roto la costilla tras el accidente de coche.

50. Sacro - (sah-crow)

Translation: Sacrum

English: The pain I have in the sacral region is due to inflammation of the sacroiliac joint.

Spanish: El dolor que tengo en la región sacra se debe a inflamación de la coyuntura sacroilíaca.

51. Esqueleto - (es-kell-etoh)

Translation: Skeleton

English: The human skeleton has bones of different shapes and sizes.

Spanish: El esqueleto humano tiene huesos de diversas formas y tamaños.

52. Cr neo, calavera - (CRAH-nay-oh, Kah-lah-ver-uh)

Translation: Skull

English: The forensic surgeon stated the marks on the cranium were caused by a blunt object.

Spanish: El forense afirmó que las marcas del cráneo se habían provocado con un objeto contundente.

53. Estern n - (es-ter-NON)

Translation: Sternum

English: The model is so skinny that her breastbone really sticks out.

Spanish: La modelo está tan delgada que se le marca mucho el esternón.

54. V rtebra - (BARE-tay-brah)

Translation: Vertebrae

English: The x-ray of his spine showed that Luis has a herniated disk between two lumbar vertebrae.

Spanish: La radiografía de la columna mostró que Luis tiene una hernia discal entre dos vértebras lumbares.

DAY 6

REPRODUCTIVE SYSTEM (FEMALE) - SISTEMA REPRODUCTIVO
FEMENINO

55. Cervix, cuello del tero/matriz - (sare-veeks, kway-yoh del OO-ter-oh)
Translation: Cervix
English: A sample was taken from the cervix for testing.
Spanish: Se tomó una muestra del cuello del útero para su análisis.

56. Trompas de Falopio - (trom-pahs day fah-loh-pee-oh)
Translation: Fallopian tube
English: The doctor told Kim that she doesn't have a cyst in her Fallopian tube.
Spanish: El médico le dijo a Kim que no tiene un quiste en la trompa de Falopio.

57. Genitales, "partes nobles", "parte femenina" - (hen-ee-tahl-uhs)
Translation: Genitals
English: Pat told his grandma that genitals do not determine gender identity.
Spanish: Pat le dijo a su abuela que los órganos genitales no determinan la identidad
de género.

58. Labia - (lah-bee-uh)
Translation: Labia

59. Cl toris - (KLEE-tor-is)
Translation: Clitoris

60. Ovarios - (oh-var-ee-ohs)

Translation: Ovaries

English: Ovaries produce estrogen and progesterone.

Spanish: Los ovarios producen el estrógeno y la progesterona.

61. tero, matriz - (OO-ter-oh, mah-treez)

Translation: Uterus

English: After birth, the uterus gradually recovers its original size.

Spanish: Después del parto, el útero recupera gradualmente su tamaño original.

62. Vulva - (bool-bah)

Translation: Vulva

63. Vagina, "la parte ntima de la mujer" - (bah-hee-nah)

Translation: Vagina

English: The gynecologist will now insert the speculum into the vagina in order to take a sample.

Spanish: Ahora el ginecólogo introducirá el espéculo en la vagina para tomar una muestra.

DAY 7

REPRODUCTIVE SYSTEM (MALE) - SISTEMA REPRODUCTIVO MASCULINO

64. Epid dimo - (Eh-pee-DEE-dee-mo)
Translation: Epididymis

65. Glande - (glahn-day)
Translation: Glans
English: My baby has a rash on his glans. What can I put on it?
Spanish: El bebé tiene una irritación en el glande. ¿Qué le puedo poner?

66. Pene, "miembro", "pip ", "pajarito", "pito (pen-ay)
Translation: Penis
English: Urine is excreted through the penis.
Spanish: La orina se excreta a través del pene.

67. Pr stata - (PRO-stah-tah)
Translation: Prostate
English: His career was cut short when he was diagnosed with prostate cancer.
Spanish: Su carrera se vio truncada cuando le diagnosticaron cáncer de próstata.

68. Escroto - (es-crow-toh)
Translation: Scrotum
English: The urologist examined the patient's scrotum and glans.
Spanish: El urólogo examinó el escroto y el glande del paciente.

69. Ves culas seminales - (bay-SEE-coo-lahs sem-ee-nahl-es)

Translation: Seminal vesicles

English: Seminal vesicle biopsy.

Spanish: Biopsia de la vesícula seminal

70. Test culos, "huevos", "bolas" - (tes-TEE-coo-los)

Translation: Testicles

English: Experiments on animals show that phthalates cause damage to the liver, kidneys and testicles.

Spanish: Se han realizado experimentos con animales que demuestran que estas sustancias producen daños en el hígado, en los riñones y en los testículos.

71. Ur ter, "ca o de la orina" - (oo-RAY-ter)

Translation: Ureter

English: Carlos underwent a procedure to dissolve the kidney stones that were obstructing his right ureter.

Spanish: Carlos se sometió a un procedimiento para disolver los cálculos que le obstruían el uréter derecho.

72. Uretra, canal - (oo-ray-trah)

Translation: Urethra

English: The pain in your urethra is due to urethritis, not a urinary tract infection.

Spanish: El dolor que siente en la uretra se debe a una uretritis, no a una infección del tracto urinario.

DAY 8

RESPIRATORY SYSTEM - SISTEMA RESPIRATORIO

73. Vias respiratorias - (bee-ahs res-peer-ah-tor-ee-ahs)
Translation: Airways
English: Avian flu to the best of my knowledge, is an infection of the gut, not of the respiratory tract.
Spanish: Que yo sepa, la gripe aviar es una infección intestinal, no de las vías respiratorias.

74. Alv olos - (al-VAY-oh-los)
Translation: Alveoli
English: Each of the lungs contains millions of alveoli.
Spanish: Cada uno de los pulmones contiene millones de alvéoli.

75. Br nquio (BROHN-kee-oh)
Translation: Bronchial tubes
English: Inflammation of the bronchial tubes is called bronchitis.
Spanish: La inflamación de los bronquios se llama bronquitis.

76. Bronquiolos - (brahn-kee-OH-los)
Translation: Bronchioles
English: The bronchioles are part of the airways in the lungs.
Spanish: Los bronquiolos son parte de las vías respiratorias en los pulmones.

77. Diafragma - (dee-ah-frahg-mah)
Translation: Diaphragm
English: You need to use your diaphragm when you sing.
Spanish: Tienes que usar el diafragma cuando cantas.

78. Pulm n, "bofe" - (pool-MOHN)

Translation: Lung

English: Smoking can have very negative effects on your lungs.

Spanish: Fumar puede tener efectos muy negativos en los pulmones.

79. Cavidad nasal, "hoyo de la nariz" - (kah-vee-dahd nahs-all)

Translation: Nasal cavity

English: The mucous in the nasal cavity is very congested.

Spanish: La mucosa de la cavidad nasal se presentaba muy congestionada.

80. Cavidad oral - (kah-vee-dahd or-all)

Translation: Oral cavity

English: The oral cavity consists of many different parts.

Spanish: La cavidad oral se compone de muchas partes distintas.

81. Tr quea - (TRAH-kee-ah)

Translation: Trachea

English: The patient was sedated and a tube was inserted into his trachea.

Spanish: El paciente fue sedado y se le introdujo un tubo en la tráquea.

DAY 9

URINARY SYSTEM - SISTEMA URINARIO

81. Vejiga - (vay-HEE-gah)
Translation: Bladder
English: She was experiencing a bladder infection.
Spanish: Tenía una infección en la vejiga.

82. Ri n - (reen-YOHN)
Translation: Kidney
English: They say that drinking lots of water is good for your kidneys.
Spanish: Dicen que beber mucha agua es bueno para los riñones.

83. Ur ter (oo-RAY-ter)
Translation: Ureter
English: Exploratory surgery revealed that both ureters were obstructed.
Spanish: Una intervención exploratoria reveló que ambos uréteres estaban obstruidos.

84. Uretra - (oo-ray-tra)
Translation: Urethra
English: The pain in your urethra is due to urethritis, not a urinary tract infection.
Spanish: El dolor que siente en la uretra se debe a una uretritis, no a una infección del tracto urinario.

SENSES - SENTIDOS

85. O do - (oh-EE-doh)
Translation: Hearing
English: His hearing has improved while his vision has declined.
Spanish: Su oído ha mejorado, mientras que su vista se ha deteriorado.

86. Vista - (bee-stah)
Translation: Vision, view
English: Ruben lost his sight due to a measles infection.
Spanish: Rubén perdió la vista debido a una infección de sarampión.

87. Olfato - (ol-fah-toh)
Translation: Smell
English: I read that smell is the most powerful of the five senses.
Spanish: Leí que el olfato es el más poderoso de los cinco sentidos.

88. Gusto - (goo-STOH)
Translation: Taste
English: Taste is one of the five senses.
Spanish: El gusto es uno de los cinco sentidos.

89. Tacto - (tahk-toh)
Translation: Touch
English: Touch is the first sense developed by a fetus.
Spanish: El primer sentido que desarrolla el feto es el tacto.

DAY 10

SIGNS & SYMPTOMS - SEÑALES Y SÍNTOMAS

90. Dolor abdominal (doh-LOHR ahb-doh-mee-nahl)
        en el est mago
        de panza/de barriga
Translation: Abdominal pain
English: He was admitted to the hospital with abdominal pain.
Spanish: Fue ingresado en el hospital con un dolor abdominal.

91. Respiraci n anormal - (res-peer-ah-see-YOHN ah-nor-mahl)
Translation: Abnormal breathing
English: The doctor checked the patient's respiration to see if she was breathing normally.
Spanish: El doctor corroboró la respiración del paciente para saber si estaba respirando normalmente.

92. Color anormal en la orina (coh-lohr ah-nor-mahl en la oh-ree-nah)
Translation: Abnormal color in the urine
English: Abnormal color in the urine could be cloudy/murky, dark or bloody.
Spanish: La orina de color anormal puede ser turbia, oscura o de color sangre.

93. Excremento (ex-kray-men-toh day ah-par-ee-en-see-uh ah-nor-mal)
heces fecales/"caca" de apariencia anormal

Translation:

Abnormal Stools:

- black	- negro
- bloody	- con sangre
- clay-colored	- de color arcilloso
- greasy	- grasiento
- hard	- duro
- loose	- suelto, aguado
- mucoid	- con moco

94. Abceso - (ahb-ses-oh)

Translation: Abscess

English: The doctor lanced the patient's abscess so it would drain.

Spanish: La doctora hizo una punción en el absceso del paciente para que se drenara.

95. Falta de menstruaci n - (fahl-tah day men-stroo-ah-see-YON)
amenorrea

Translation: Absent period, amenorrhea

English: The absence of a woman's monthly menstrual period is called amenorrhea.

Spanish: La ausencia de los períodos menstruales mensuales de una mujer se llama amenorrea.

96. Acné, barros, espinillas, granos - (ack-NAY)

Translation: Acne

English: She buys medication to fight acne at the first sight of a pimple.

Spanish: Compra medicamentos para el acné a la primera señal de espinillas.

97. Adenoiditis - (Ah-den-oh-ee-dee-tis)

Translation: Adenoiditis

English: Adenoiditis is the inflammation of the adenoid tissue, usually caused by an infection.

Spanish: La adenoiditis es una inflamación, generalmente producida por una infección de las adenoides.

98. Agitado - (ah-hee-tah-doh)

Translation: Agitated

English: The patient's breathing was rapid so he was given a sedative.

Spanish: La respiración del paciente estaba agitada así que le dieron un calmante.

99. Alergia - (ah-LAIR-hee-ah)

Translation: Allergy

English: It seems there are more and more children suffering from peanut allergy these days.

Spanish: Parece que cada día hay más niños que sufren de alergia al maní.

100. Ansiedad - (ahn-see-ay-dahd)

Translation: Anxiety

English: Money is a constant source of worry for me.

Spanish: El dinero es una fuente constante de ansiedad.

DAY 11

SIGNS & SYMPTOMS - SEÑALES Y SÍNTOMAS

101. Anemia "sangre delgada" (ah-nay-mee-uh, sahn-grey del-gah-da)
"debilidad de la sangre"
"falta de sangre"
Translation: Anemia

English: Her anemia causes her to feel tired and dizzy.

Spanish: La anemia hace que se sienta fatigada y mareada.

102. Rabia (rah-bee-ah)
Translation: Anger

English: The man was filled with anger when he saw that someone had scratched his car.

Spanish: El hombre se llenó de rabia cuando vio que alguien había rayado su carro.

103. Apat a - (ah-pah-TEE-ah)
Translation: Apathy

English: The level of corruption in the government has produced much apathy among the electorate.

Spanish: El nivel de corrupción en el gobierno ha producido mucha apatía entre el electorado.

104. Apendicitis (ah-pen-dee-see-tus)
Translation: Appendicitis

English: My appendicitis was so severe that I had to get my appendix removed immediately.

Spanish: Mi apendicitis era tan severa que tuvieron que quitarme el apéndice inmediatamente.

105. Artritis - (ar-tree-tus)
Translation: Arthritis
English: The arthritis in his hands prevents him from playing the guitar.
Spanish: La artritis que tiene en las manos le impide tocar la guitarra.

106. Asfixia, sofocaci n - (aus-fix-ee-uh, sof-oh-kah-see-YOHN)
Translation: Asphyxia, Suffocation
English: The small parts of the toy can cause the asphyxiation of young children.
Spanish: Las piezas pequeñas del juguete pueden provocar la asfixia de los niños pequeños.

107. Pie de atleta - (pee-ay day at-let-ah)
Translation: Athlete's foot
English: Preventing athlete's foot can be difficult, but keeping your feet clean and dry will help.
Spanish: Prevenir el pie de atleta puede resultar difícil, pero mantener sus pies limpios y secos ayudará.

108. Atrofia muscular - (ah-troh-fee-ah moo-skoo-lar)
Translation: Muscular atrophy
English: In most people, muscle atrophy is caused by not using the muscles enough.
Spanish: En la mayoría de las personas, la atrofia muscular es causada por no utilizar los músculos lo suficiente.

109. Dolor de espalda - (doh-lor day es-pahl-dah)

Translation: Backache

English: The patient said she had suffered a backache for over a week.

Spanish: La paciente dijo que había tenido dolor de espalda desde hacía una semana.

110. Mal aliento, halitosis - (mahl ah-lee-en-toh, ah-lee-toh-sees)

Translation: Bad breath, halitosis

English: Don't get any closer. I've eaten some onion and have very bad breath.

Spanish: No te acerques. He comido cebolla y tengo muy mal aliento.

111. Calvo - (kahl-voh)

Translation: Bald

English: At thirty he was already going bald, so he decided to shave his head.

Spanish: A los 30 años ya se estaba quedando calvo, así que decidió raparse la cabeza.

112. Eructo - (eh-rooc-toh)

Translation: Burp/belch

English: In some cultures, a burp is a compliment. It means the diner enjoyed the meal.

Spanish: En algunas culturas, el eructo representa un elogio. Significa que el comensal disfrutó la comida.

DAY 12

SIGNS & SYMPTOMS - SEÑALES Y SÍNTOMAS

113. Espinillas (es-pee-nee-yas)
Translation: Blackheads
English: Some degree of acne is seen in 85% of adolescents, and nearly all teens have the occasional pimple, blackhead, or whitehead.
Spanish: Se observa cierto grado de acné en el 85% de los adolescentes y casi todos tienen el grano esporádico, espinillas o puntos blancos.

114. Sangrar (sahn-grar)
Translation: To Bleed
English: The nurse pricked my finger and it started to bleed.
Spanish: La enfermera me pinchó el dedo y este empezó a sangrar.

115. Sangrar entre per odos/reglas - (sahn-grar en-tray pair-EE-oh-dos/ray-glas)
Translation: Bleeding between periods
English: Menstrual pain and bleeding, as well as bleeding between periods, are increased with the copper IUD, but decreased with the hormonal IUD.
Spanish: El dolor y sangrado menstrual, así como el sangrado entre períodos, aumentan con el DIU de cobre, pero disminuyen con el DIU hormonal.

116. Mancha (mahn-cha)
Translation: blemish/stain
English: If a finding or spot seems suspicious, your radiologist may recommend further diagnostic studies.
Spanish: Si un resultado o una mancha resultan sospechosos, su radiólogo puede recomendarle estudios de diagnóstico adicionales.

117. Ceguera - (say-gare-uh)
Translation: Blindness
English: His blindness didn't stop him from learning to play the piano.
Spanish: Su ceguera no le impidió aprender a tocar el piano.

118. Ampolla, vejiga - (am-poy-ya, vay-hee-gah)
Translation: Blister
English: Opening the blister increases the chance of infection and delays healing.
Spanish: Abrir la ampolla aumenta la probabilidad de infección y retrasa la curación.

119. Hinchado, distendido - (een-cha-doh, dis-ten-dee-doh)
Translation: Bloated / swollen
English: Elena's finger was so swollen that she couldn't get her ring off.
Spanish: A Elena se le había hinchado tanto el dedo que no podía quitarse el anillo.

120. Co gulo de sangre - (koh-AH-goo-loh day sahn-grey)
Translation: Blood clot
English: A blood clot can break free in the leg and travel to the lungs (pulmonary embolus) or anywhere else in the body, and can be life threatening.
Spanish: Un coágulo de sangre se puede desprender de la pierna y viajar a los pulmones (émbolo pulmonar) o a cualquiera otra parte en el cuerpo y es potencialmente mortal.

121. Flujo de sangre - (floo-ho day sahn-grey)
Translation: Blood flow
English: Symptoms usually do not occur until blood flow becomes slowed or blocked.
Spanish: Los síntomas generalmente no se presentan hasta que el flujo de sangre se vuelve lento o resulta obstruido.

122. Sangre en el esputo/flema - (sahn-grey en el es-poo-toh, flem-ah)
Translation: Blood in sputum
English: Fever, increased coughing, changes in sputum or blood in sputum, loss of appetite, or other signs of pneumonia.
Spanish: Fiebre, aumento de la tos, cambios en el esputo o sangre en el esputo, inapetencia u otros signos de neumonía.

123. Piel azulada, cianosis, "ponerse morado" - (pee-ehl ah-zoo-lah-dah)
Translation: Bluish skin, cyanosis
English: Wheezing occurs with significant shortness of breath, bluish skin, confusion, or mental status changes.
Spanish: Las sibilancias ocurren con una significativa falta de respiración, piel azulada, confusión o cambios en el estado mental.

124. Vista nublada/empa ada - (vee-stah nu-blah-dah/em-pahn-yah-dah)
Translation: Cloudy/blurred vision
English: Cloudy vision can also come about in the presence of other medical conditions, some of which are very serious.
Spanish: La vista nublada también puede manifestarse en presencia de otras patologías médicas, algunas de las cuales son muy graves.

125. Grano, comed n - (grah-noh, koh-may-DOHN)
Translation: Boil, pimple
English: The basic acne lesion is called a boil.
Spanish: La lesión básica producida por el acné se denomina comedón.

DAY 13

126. Deformidad de los huesos (day-form-ee-dahd day los way-sohs)

Translation: Bone deformity

English: Clubfoot is a common deformity of the bones and joints in the foot that is seen in newborns.

Spanish: El pie equinovaro es una deformidad común de los huesos y coyunturas.

127. Fractura/quebradura de los huesos (frahk-too-rah/kay-brah-doo-rah day los way-sohs)

Translation: Bone fracture

English: Having strong bones helps prevent osteoporosis and bone fractures later in life.

Spanish: El tener huesos fuertes ayuda a prevenir la osteoporosis y las fracturas de los huesos en la edad avanzada.

128. Sangre en la orina - (sahn-grey en lah oh-ree-nah)

Translation: Blood in the urine

English: The first symptoms of nephritis usually are high levels of protein and blood in the urine.

Spanish: Los primeros síntomas de la nefritis son niveles altos de proteína y sangre en la orina.

129. Presi n arterial, tensi n (pres-ee-YON ar-tare-ree-all)

Translation: Blood pressure

        - low   - baja
        - high   - alta

English: This is a healthy diet plan that helps control blood pressure.

Spanish: Éste es un plan de alimentación saludable que ayuda a controlar la presión arterial.

130. Piernas arqueadas, "patizambo", cascorvo - (pee-air-nahs ar-kay-ah-dahs)

Translation: Arched legs, bow-legged

English: Children are naturally bow-legged until the age of three.

Spanish: Los niños son naturalmente piernas arqueadas hasta la edad de tres años.

131. Derrame/embolia cerebral - (Day-rrah-may/em-boh-lee-ah ser-ray-brahl)

Translation: Brain stroke

English: A brain hemorrhage paralyzed his body's left side.

Spanish: Un derrame cerebral le paralizó el lado izquierdo del cuerpo.

132. Bronquitis - (brohn-kee-tus)

Translation: Bronquitis

English: If bronchitis is caught early enough, you can prevent the damage to your lungs.

Spanish: Si la bronquitis se detecta de manera oportuna, se puede prevenir el daño a los pulmones.

133. Moret n, morado, cardenal, magulladura - (moh-ray-TOHN)

Translation: Bruise

English: What causes bruising and internal damage to the brain?

Spanish: ¿Cuál es la causa de los moretones y del daño interno en el encéfalo?

134. Chich n - (chee-CHONE)

Translation: Bump

English: The area may be tender to touch and a bump at the treatment site may be noticeable.

Spanish: El área podrá ser blanda al tacto y podrá notarse un chichón en el área del tratamiento.

135. Juanetes - (wah-net-es)

Translation: Bunions

English: You should check your feet everyday for calluses, bunions, sores, or discolored skin.

Spanish: Revise sus pies todos los días para ver si tiene callos, juanetes, llagas o manchas en la piel.

DAY 14

136. Quemadura (kay-mah-doo-rah)
Translation: Burn
English: Keep your child out of the sun until the burn is healed.
Spanish: Mantenga a su hijo alejado del sol hasta que se haya curado la quemadura.

137. Sensaci n de ardor, "quemaz n" (sen-sah-SYON day ar-dor)
Translation: Burning feeling
English: You may feel a burning sensation when the area is anesthetized.
Spanish: Puede sentir una sensación de ardor en el área cuando se aplica la anestesia.

138. Bursitis - (boor-see-tis)
Translation: Bursitis
English: The treatment of any bursitis depends on whether or not it involves infection.
Spanish: El tratamiento de la bursitis depende de si existe o no una infección.

139. P rdida de calcio (PARE-dee-dah day kal-see-yoh)
Translation: Calcium loss
English: Cutting back on caffeine and alcohol may reduce symptoms of anxiety, insomnia, and loss of calcium.
Spanish: Consumir menos cafeína y alcohol puede aliviar los síntomas de ansiedad, insomnio y pérdida de calcio.

140. Paro card aco, ataque al coraz n, paro del coraz n - (Pa-roh kar-dee-ack-oh, ah-tack-ay al cor-ah-ZONE)
Translation: Cardiac arrest
English: The doctors suspect a heart attack to be the cause behind this unfortunate incident.
Spanish: Los médicos sospechan que la causa del fallecimiento fue un paro cardíaco.

141. Arritmia card aca - (ah-rrit-mee-ah kar-dee-ack-ah)
Translation: Cardiac arrhythmia
English: Atrial fibrillation is the most common sustained arrhythmia.
Spanish: La fibrilación auricular es la arritmia cardíaca sostenida más frecuente.

142. Par lisis cerebral - (pah-RAHL-ee-sees ser-ay-brahl)
Translation: Cerebral palsy
English: Cerebral palsy is caused by injuries or abnormalities of the brain.
Spanish: La parálisis cerebral es causada por lesiones o anomalías del cerebro.

143. Labios resecos/partidos/agrietados - (lah-bee-yohs ray-sek-ohs)
Translation: Chapped lips
English: Dry skin and lips--your doctor can suggest lotions or creams to use.
Spanish: Piel y labios resecos: su médico le puede sugerir cremas y lociones para usar.

144. Saba n - (sah-bahn-nYON)
Translation: Chilblain
English: People with poor circulation are more likely to get chilblains.
Spanish: Las personas con mala circulación tienen más probabilidades de presentar sabañón.

145. Atragantarse, atorarse - (ah-trah-gahn-tar-say, ah-toh-rar-say)

Translation: To choke

English: Children younger than 5 years can easily choke on food and small objects.

Spanish: Un niño menor de cinco años puede atragantarse fácilmente con alimentos y objetos pequeños.

DAY 15

146. Circuncisi n (seer-koon-sis-ee-YON)
Translation: Circumcision
English: Your baby's physician will give you specific instructions on the care of the circumcision.
Spanish: El médico de su bebé le dará instrucciones específicas sobre el cuidado de la circuncisión.

147. Labio leporino (lah-bee-yoh lep-or-ee-noh)
Translation: Cleft lip, harelip
English: The exact cause of cleft lip and cleft palate is not completely understood.
Spanish: La causa exacta del labio leporino y del paladar hendido no se conoce completamente.

148. Bursitis - (bur-see-tis)
Translation: Bursitis
English: The treatment of any bursitis depends on whether or not it involves infection.
Spanish: El tratamiento de la bursitis depende de si existe o no una infección.

149. Coagulaci n de la sangre (coh-ah-goo-lah-SYON day la sahn-grey)
Translation: Clotting of blood
English: Medications that help to prevent additional blood clots from forming are called anticoagulants, as they prevent the coagulation of the blood.
Spanish: Los medicamentos que ayudan a evitar que se formen más coágulos de sangre se llaman anticoagulantes, ya que impiden la coagulación de la sangre.

150. Lengua pastosa - (len-gwah pah-stoh-sah)
Translation: Coated tongue

English: Her mouth was dry, her tongue coated, and she always had to drink sparkling mineral water, because her lips were dry and [...] the saliva was white and sticky.

Spanish: Tenía la boca seca, la lengua pastosa, y tenía que beber continuamente agua mineral ya que sus labios estaban secos y la saliva era blanca y pegajosa.

151. Catarro, resfriado, gripa, gripe - (kah-tah-rroh, res-free-ah-doh)
Translation: Cold, flu

English: If you have a cold, the flu, or other viral illness, drink plenty of fluids to prevent getting dehydrated.

Spanish: Si la persona tiene un resfriado, gripe o cualquier otra enfermedad viral, debe tomar muchos líquidos para prevenir la deshidratación.

152. Piel fr a - (pee-ehl FREE-ah)
Translation: Cold skin

English: Symptoms include pain in the legs or feet, clammy cool skin, and a diminished sense of heat and cold.

Spanish: Entre los síntomas se incluyen dolor en las piernas o los pies, piel fría y húmeda, y una disminución de la sensibilidad al frío y al calor.

153. Frialdad de manos y pies/extremidades - (free-ahl-ee-dahd day mah-nos ee pee-ays)
Translation: Coldness in extremities

English: Sometimes, beta blockers can make your hands and feet especially cold.

Spanish: En ocaciones, los betabloqueantes pueden producir una intensa frialdad de las manos y los pies.

154. Cólico, "retorsijón", "retortijón", "torzón" - (KOH-lee-koh)
Translation: Colic

English: The colic may start in the afternoon and may last several hours; then, it suddenly disappears.

Spanish: El cólico suele empezar por la tarde y puede durar varias horas, después se le pasa de repente.

155. Colapso - (koh-laps-oh)
Translation: Collapse

English: How well a person does after having a collapsed lung depends on what caused it.

Spanish: El pronóstico de una persona después de tener un colapso pulmonar depende de lo que lo causó.

DAY 16

SIGNS & SYMPTOMS - SEÑALES Y SÍNTOMAS

156. Coma (koh-mah)
Translation: Coma
English: If it is not treated correctly, cryptococcal meningitis can cause coma or death.
Spanish: Si no se trata correctamente, la meningitis criptocócica puede provocar el coma o la muerte.

157. Quejarse (kay-har-say)
Translation: To complain
English: When the child regains consciousness, the child may complain of being tired or sleepy after the seizure.
Spanish: Cuando el niño vuelve en sí después de la convulsión puede quejarse de sentirse cansado o somnoliento.

158. Congesti n - (kon-hest-ee-YOHN)
Translation: Congestion
English: It helps loosen congestion in your chest and throat, making it easier to cough out through your mouth.
Spanish: Se usa para aliviar la congestión y la mucosidad para ayudarlo respirar más fácil.

159. Estre imiento (es-treh-nyee-me-en-toh)
Translation: Constipation
English: Stress and travel can also contribute to constipation or other changes in bowel habits.
Spanish: El estrés y los viajes también pueden contribuir al estreñimiento u otros cambios en las deposiciones.

160. Contracciones (kon-trak-see-ohn-es)

Translation: Contractions

English: Regularity of any contractions will also be monitored, and an ultrasound may be performed.

Spanish: También se revisará la regularidad de las contracciones, y se puede realizar un ultrasonido.

161. Convulsiones, "ataques", "chiripioca" - (kon-vuhl-see-yohn-es)

Translation: Convulsions/seizures

English: The health care provider will do a physical exam and rule out other possible causes of seizures.

Spanish: El médico llevará a cabo un examen físico y descartará otras posibles causas de las convulsiones.

162. Callo - (kah-yo)

Translation: Corn/callus

English: If you suspect that your corn or callus is infected or is not getting better despite treatment, contact your health care provider.

Spanish: Si sospecha que una callosidad o un callo está infectado o no está mejorando a pesar del tratamiento, contacte al médico.

163. Tos - (Tohs)

Translation: Cough

English: The doctor prescribed me a syrup for my cough.

Spanish: El doctor me recetó un jarabe para la tos.

164. Expectoraci n de sangre, tos con sangre - (ex-pek-tor-ah-SYOHN day sahn-grey)

Translation: Coughing up blood

English: Are you coughing up large amounts of blood (massive hemoptysis)?

Spanish: ¿Está expectorando grandes cantidades de sangre (hemoptisis masiva)?

165. Calambre, cólico, "retortijón", "torzón" - (kah-lahm-bray)
Translation: Cramp
English: The biopsy sampling causes little or no pain, although you may have some mild cramping.
Spanish: La muestra para la biopsia causa poco o ningún dolor, aunque usted puede sentir un leve calambre.

DAY 17

176. Estrabismo, bizco, "bizquera" (es-trah-bees-moh)
Translation: Cross-eye/strabismus
English: The onset of strabismus is most common in children younger than 6 years of age.
Spanish: La aparición del estrabismo es más frecuente en los niños menores de 6 años de edad.

177. Costra, escara (koh-strah)
Translation: Crust, scab
English: Cover with a bandage and change it every day until a scab forms.
Spanish: Cúbrala con un vendaje y cámbielo todos los días hasta que se forme costra.

178. Cortada, herida - (kor-tah-dah)
Translation: cut/wound
English: That is why it is very important to monitor the wound daily.
Spanish: Por ello es muy importante controlar la herida a diario.

179. Quiste, "bolita", "pelotita" (kee-stay)
Translation: Cyst
English: This procedure involves guiding a very fine needle into the cyst and drawing fluid from it.
Spanish: Este procedimiento incluye el guiar una aguja fina dentro del quiste y el extraer fluido del mismo.

180. Caspa - (kahs-pah)

Translation: Dandruff

English: Treatment usually includes the use of dandruff shampoo on the skin, as prescribed by your physician.

Spanish: El tratamiento suele incluir la aplicación de champú para la caspa sobre la piel, según lo indique el médico.

181. Sordera - (sor-dare-uh)

Translation: Deafness

English: Which design will work best for my type of hearing loss?

Spanish: ¿Qué modelo funcionará mejor para mi tipo de sordera?

182. Deformidad, deformaci n - (day-for-mee-dahd, deh-for-mah-SYOHN)

Translation: Deformity

English: Be sure to consult your child's physician if there is a prolonged, visible deformity of the affected area.

Spanish: Asegúrese de consultar con el médico de su hijo si hay una deformidad visible y prolongada de la zona afectada.

183. Deshidrataci n, "estar seco" - (des-ee-drah-tah-SYOHN)

Translation: Dehydration

English: Dehydration can be very serious, even life threatening if body fluids are dangerously low.

Spanish: La deshidratación puede ser muy grave y hasta volverse un peligro de muerte si la cantidad de líquido del cuerpo baja demasiado.

184. Deca do(a) - (day-kye-EE-doh/dah)

Translation: Decayed/deteriorated

English: Unfortunately, the situation has significantly deteriorated over the past year.

Spanish: Lamentablemente, la situación se ha deteriorado considerablemente durante el año transcurrido.

185. Delirio - (deh-leer-ee-oh)

Translation: Delirium

English: Some theories affirm that during delirium the level of psychic activity is reduced.

Spanish: Hay teorías que afirman que durante el delirio se baja el nivel de la vida psíquica.

DAY 18

186. Deprimido(a) (deh-pre-me-doh/dah)
Translation: Depressed
English: If you wonder whether your child might be depressed, it's worth bringing to a doctor's attention.
Spanish: Si los padres creen que su hijo podría estar deprimido, vale la pena consultarlo con el médico.

187. Depresi n (deh-pres-SYON)
Translation: Depression
English: Smoking has been associated with depression and psychological distress
Spanish: El fumar se ha asociado con la depresión y con los trastornos psicológicos.

188. Dermatitis - (der-mah-tee-tis)
Translation: Dermatitis
English: The most common cause of eczema is atopic dermatitis, sometimes called infantile eczema although it occurs in infants and older children.
Spanish: La causa más habitual del eccema es la dermatitis atópica, a veces denominada eccema del lactante, aunque puede afectar tanto a lactantes como a niños mayores.

189. Diarrea (dee-ah-rray-ah)
Translation: Diarrhea
English: One of the biggest threats is the outbreak of water-borne diseases such as cholera and diarrhea.
Spanish: Una de las más graves amenazas es el brote de enfermedades transmitidas por el agua como el cólera y la diarrea.

190. Dificultad al tragar/pasar - (dif-ee-kul-tahd al trah-gar/pah-sar)

Translation: Difficulty in swallowing

English: If you experience chest pain, vomiting or difficulty in swallowing or breathing after taking this product, seek immediate medical attention.

Spanish: Si experimenta dolor de pecho, vómitos, dificultad al tragar o respirar luego de la toma del producto, consulte inmediatamente a un médico.

191. Pupila dilatada - (pu-PEE-lah dee-lah-tah-dah)

Translation: Dilated pupil

English: After the initial exam, he said, a dilated eye exam is needed every year thereafter.

Spanish: Luego del examen inicial, dijo, la prueba de pupila dilatada es necesaria cada año.

192. Supuraci n, secreci n, descarga, "desecho" - (su-pu-rah-SYON)

Translation: Discharge

English: Any inflammation or oozing/discharge should always be reported immediately to the physician.

Spanish: Cualquier inflamación o supuración siempre debe informarse de inmediato al médico.

193. Molestia - (moh-les-tee-ah)

Translation: Discomfort

English: Stable angina is chest pain or discomfort that typically occurs with activity or stress.

Spanish: Es una molestia o dolor torácico que clásicamente ocurre con actividad o estrés.

194. Enfermedad, dolencia - (en-fer-may-dahd, doh-len-see-ah)

Translation: Disease, illness

English: Cigarette smoking produces a greater risk for coronary heart disease in people younger than 50 years of age.

Spanish: Fumar cigarrillos produce un riesgo mayor de enfermedad coronaria en las persones menores de 50 años.

195. Desfiguraci n - (des-fig-oo-rah-SYON)

Translation: Disfigurement

English: Plastic surgery may be needed to correct the disfigurement caused by sores on the face.

Spanish: Puede necesitarse una cirugía plástica para corregir la desfiguración causada por las llagas en la cara.

DAY 19

196. Dislocaci n, descoyuntura, desencaje, zafadura, recalcada (dees-loh-kah-SYOHN)
Translation: Dislocation
English: A dislocation occurs when extreme force is put on a ligament, allowing the ends of two connected bones to separate.
Spanish: Una dislocación se produce cuando al aplicar una fuerza extrema sobre un ligamento se separan los dos extremos del hueso.

197. Mareo, v rtigo (mah-ray-oh)
Translation: Dizziness
English: Did another illness develop before or after the dizziness began?
Spanish: ¿Se desarrolló alguna otra enfermedad después que comenzó el mareo?

198. Visi n doble, "ver doble" - (vis-ee-YOHN doh-blay)
Translation: Double vision
English: There can also be problems with walking and coordination, as well as double vision.
Spanish: También se pueden originar dificultades en la marcha y la coordinación, así como visión doble.

199. Goteo (go-tay-oh)
Translation: Drip
English: It could be given through injections or via an intravenous drip, he said.
Spanish: Podría ser administrada con inyecciones o con goteo intravenoso, dijo.

200. Somnolencia, amodorramiento, adormecimiento - (som-noh-len-see-ah)

Translation: Drowsiness

English: What have you done to try to relieve the drowsiness?

Spanish: ¿Qué ha hecho para tratar de aliviar la somnolencia?

201. Tos seca - (tohs sek-ah)

Translation: Dry cough

English: A chronic dry cough may be a sign of mild asthma.

Spanish: Una tos seca crónica puede ser un signo de asma leve.

202. Boca seca - (boh-kah sek-ah)

Translation: Dry mouth

English: The most common side effects of these medicines are dry mouth and constipation.

Spanish: Los efectos secundarios de estos medicamentos son boca seca y estreñimiento.

203. Piel seca - (pee-ehl sek-ah)

Translation: Dry skin

English: Do not apply this medicine to sunburned, windburned, dry, chapped, irritated, or broken skin.

Spanish: No aplique esta medicina a la piel quemada por el sol, el viento, piel seca, quebrada, irritada, o abierta.

204. Disenter a, "pujos" - (dee-sen-tare-EE-ah)

Translation: Dysentery

English: Contact your doctor if you think you may have amoebic dysentery.

Spanish: Consulte a su médico si cree que puede tener disentería amebiana.

205. Dispepsia - (dees-pep-see-ah)

Translation: Dyspepsia

English: For treatment of dyspepsia, cayenne may be taken at a dosage of 0.5 to 1.0 g three times daily (prior to meals).

Spanish: Para el tratamiento de la dispepsia, el pimiento de cayena podría tomarse a una dosis de 0.5 a 1.0 gramos tres veces al día (antes de las comidas).

DAY 20

SIGNS & SYMPTOMS - SEÑALES Y SÍNTOMAS

206. Infecci n de o do (in-fek-SYOHN day oh-EE-doh)
Translation: Ear infection
English: By the age of 3, more than 80 percent of children have had at least one ear infection.
Spanish: Para los 3 años, más del 80 por ciento de los niños han tenido al menos una infección de oído.

207. Dolor de o do (doh-lor day oh-EE-doh)
Translation: Ear ache
English: How do I know if my child has an earache?
Spanish: ¿Cómo sé si mi hijo tiene dolor de oídos?

208. Eczema - (ek-zeh-ma)
Translation: Eczema
English: The symptoms of eczema can vary from person to person.
Spanish: Los síntomas del eccema varían de una persona a otra.

209. Edema, "hinchado", "inflamado" (eh-dem-ah)
Translation: Edema
English: Swelling of the ankles, hands, and face may occur (called edema), as the mother continues to retain fluids.
Spanish: Posible hinchazón de los tobillos, manos y cara (denominada edema) causada por la retención de fluidos por parte de la madre.

210. Epididimitis - (eh-pee-dee-dee-mee-tis)
Translation: Epididymitis
English: Epididymitis is usually caused by the spread of an infection from the urethra or the bladder.
Spanish: La epididimitis generalmente es causada por la diseminación de una infección desde la uretra o la vejiga.

211. Dificultad en la erecci n - (dif-ee-kul-tahd en la eh-rrek-SYOHN)
Translation: Erection difficulties
English: Antidepressants can have numerous effects on sexual function including altered sexual desire, erection difficulties and orgasm problems.
Spanish: Los antidepresivos pueden tener numerosos efectos en la función sexual, que incluyen la alteración del deseo sexual, las dificultades en la erección y los problemas con el orgasmo

212. Erupci n, ronchas - (eh-roop-SYOHN)
Translation: Rash, eruption
English: Your doctor may give you an antihistamine medication to help relieve the rash.
Spanish: Es posible que su médico le administre un medicamento antihistamínico para ayudar a aliviar la erupción cutánea.

213. Euforia, excitaci n - (eh-oo-for-ee-ah)
Translation: Euphoria
English: I felt pure joy and elation when I first saw them!
Spanish: Sentí pura alegría y euforia cuando los vi por primera vez!

214. Dolor excesivo durante la menstruaci n/regla -
(doh-lor ex-ses-see-voh dur-ahn-tay la men-stroo-ah-SYOHN)
Translation: Excessive pain during period
English: Although some pain during menstruation is normal, excessive pain is not.
Spanish: Aunque algo de dolor durante la menstruación es normal, el dolor
excesivo no lo es.

215. Salivaci n excesiva, mucha saliva - (sah-lee-vah-SYOHN ex-ses-see-vah)
Translation: Excessive salivation
English: Avoid excessive salivation.
Spanish: Evite el exceso de salivación.

DAY 21

216. Agotamiento, fatiga, cansancio excesivo (ah-go-tah-mee-en-toh, fah-tee-ga)
Translation: Exhaustion, fatigue
English: All other possible causes of fatigue are eliminated before this diagnosis is made.
Spanish: Se descartan primero todas las otras causas de fatiga antes de este diagnóstico.

217. Desmayo (des-my-oh)
Translation: Fainting
English: Does fainting occur when you change positions -- for example, go from lying to standing?
Spanish: ¿El desmayo ocurre cuando cambia de posiciones, por ejemplo, estar acostado y luego pararse?

218. Cloasma, pa o, manchas en la cara - (kloh-ahs-mah)
Translation: Chloasma
English: Up to 70 percent of pregnant women develop chloasma.
Spanish: Hasta un 70 por ciento de las mujeres embarazadas presentarán cloasma.

219. Par lisis de la cara (pa-RAH-lee-sis day la kah-rah)
Translation: Facial paralysis
English: Like brain surgery, radiosurgery can sometimes result in paralysis of the face or loss of hearing.
Spanish: Al igual que la cirugía cerebral, la radiocirugía algunas veces puede provocar parálisis de la cara o pérdida de la audición.

220. Fatiga, cansancio - (fah-TEE-gah, kan-sahn-see-yo)

Translation: Fatigue

English: Lack of sleep can cause fatigue.

Spanish: La falta de sueño puede causar fatiga.

221. Fiebre, "calentura", "temperatura", "estar ardiendo" - (fee-ay-bray, kal-en-toor-ah)

Translation: Fever

English: You can ask your mom or dad to give you a pain reliever if you have a fever or if your muscles are sore.

Spanish: Puedes pedirle a tu mamá o a tu papá que te den una medicina para aliviar el dolor o la fiebre, si tienes fiebre o si te duelen los músculos.

222. Llagas de fiebre, fuegos, "fogazos" - (yah-gahs day fee-ay-bray, fway-gohs)

Translation: Fever blisters

English: Fever, sore throat, or mouth sores last for more than 5 days.

Spanish: La fiebre, el dolor de garganta o las llagas en la boca persisten por más de 5 días.

223. Fibroide, fibroma - (fee-bro-ee-day, fee-bro-mah)

Translation: Fibroid

English: Rarely, a large fibroid can block the opening of the uterus or keep the baby from passing into the birth canal.

Spanish: En raras ocasiones, un fibroma grande puede bloquear la abertura del útero o no permitir que el bebé pase por el canal de parto.

224. Pie plano - (pee-ay plah-no)

Translation: Flatfoot

English: Flat foot is a defect of your foot that eliminates the arch.

Spanish: Un pie plano es un defecto de su pie que elimina el arco.

225. Ruborizarse, sonrojarse, "ponerse colorado", "chiviado" - (ru-bori-sar-say, son-roh-har-say)

Translation: To blush

English: A tendency to flush or blush easily.

Spanish: Tendencia a sonrojarse o ruborizarse con facilidad.

DAY 22

SIGNS & SYMPTOMS - SEÑALES Y SÍNTOMAS

226. Pecas (pek-ahs)
Translation: Freckles
English: Exposure to sunlight increases the production of melanin, which is why people get suntanned or freckled.
Spanish: La exposición a la luz solar aumenta la producción de melanina, razón por la cual las personas se broncean o desarrollan pecas.

227. Frigidez (frih-hee-des)
Translation: Frigidity
English: Stress is known to have a negative effect on sexual functions, libido, frigidity, fertility, sperm count and mobility, symptoms of menopause, andropause, PMS, etc.
Spanish: El estrés tiene igualmente un efecto negativo sobre la función sexual, el libido, frigidez, fertilidad, conteo y motilidad del esperma, síntomas de la menopausia, andropausia, SPM, etc.

228. Inquieto(a), molesto(a) - (en-kee-eh-toh/tah)
Translation: Fussy/restless
English: He's a restless and vivacious child.
Spanish: Es un niño inquieto y vivaracho.

229. C lculos/piedas renales, "piedras en la hiel" (CAL-koo-los/pee-ay-drahs ray-nahl-es)
Translation: Gallstones/kidney stones
English: If the crystals build up in the kidneys, kidney stones may result.
Spanish: Si los cristales se acumulan en los riñones, se pueden producir cálculos renales.

230. Gastritis - (gas-tree-tis)
Translation: Gastritis

English: Coffee can help in the disease-fighting process, but it allegedly may also be linked with osteoporosis and gastritis.

Spanish: El café puede ayudar en el proceso de combatir la enfermedad, pero podría también estar ligado a osteoporosis y gastritis.

231. Bocio, "buche", "g eg echo" - (fee-ay-bray, kal-en-toor-ah)
Translation: Goiter/goitre

English: The cause of toxic nodular goiter is not known.

Spanish: La causa del bocio nodular tóxico no se conoce.

232. Dolores de crecimiento - (doh-lore-es day cres-ee-mee-en-toh)
Translation: Growing pains

English: It is common for young people in this age group to experience actual, physical growing pains.

Spanish: Es común para los jóvenes de esta edad experimentar dolores de crecimiento físicos reales.

233. Alucinar, "estar mal de la cabeza" - (ah-lu-see-nar)
Translation: Hallucinate

English: A person who begins to hallucinate and is detached from reality should get checked by a health care professional right away.

Spanish: Una persona que empieza a alucinar y se separa de la realidad debe ser evaluada de inmediato por un profesional de la salud.

234. N dulos endurecidos - (NOH-du-lohs)
Translation: Hard nodules/lump

English: They can help you know if you have a hardened lump or other change in your breast that you should get checked out.

Spanish: Pueden ayudarla a saber si hay nódulos endurecidos o cualquier otra alteración en los senos que deba ser revisada.

235. Fiebre de heno, romadizo - (fee-ay-bray day ay-noh, roh-mah-dee-zoh)
Translation: Hay fever

English: Hives are a common reaction, especially in people with other allergies like hay fever.

Spanish: La urticaria es una reacción común, especialmente en las personas con otras reacciones alérgicas, como la fiebre de heno.

DAY 23

236. Dolor de cabeza, jaqueca, "chontal" (doh-lohr day kah-bay-sah)
Translation: Headache
English: We need to look at what is causing the headache.
Spanish: Tenemos que averiguar lo que causa ese dolor de cabeza.

237. P rdida del o do, p rdida de la audici n, "quedarse sordo" (PARE-dee-dah del oh-EE-doh)
Translation: Hearing loss
English: Loss of hearing is clearly the most widely-known harmful effect of noise.
Spanish: La pérdida del oído es la consecuencia desfavorable más conocida que causa el ruido.

238. Ataque al coraz n, infarto - (ah-tak-ay all kor-ah-SOHN, en-far-toh)
Translation: Heart attack
English: You should not use this medication if you have had a heart attack.
Spanish: Usted no debe usar esta medicina si ha tenido un ataque al corazón.

239. Soplo/murmullo del coraz n (soh-ploh/moor-moo-yoh del kor-ah-SOHN)
Translation: Heart murmur
English: Have you ever been told you have a heart murmur?
Spanish: ¿Le han dicho alguna vez que tiene murmullo en el corazón?

240. Latido del coraz n - (lah-tee-doh del kor-ah-SOHN)
Translation: Heartbeat

- extra   - extra
- fast   - rápido
- irregular   - irregular
- skipped   - intermitente
- slow   - lento

English: The process is repeated with each heart beat.
Spanish: Este proceso se repite con cada latido del corazón.

241. Acidez estomacal, aced a, agruras, agriura, agrieras, "fogazo" - (ah-see-des es-toh-mah-kal)
Translation: Heartburn/stomach acid
English: About 50% of pregnant women have heartburn in the third trimester.
Spanish: Aproximadamente el 50% de mujeres embarazadas tienen acidez estomacal en el tercer trimestre.

242. Hemorragia, desangramiento - (em-oh-rrah-hee-ah, day-sahn-gra-mee-en-toh)
Translation: Hemorrhage
English: As with all surgeries, there is a risk for heavy bleeding.
Spanish: Como con todas las cirugías, hay un riesgo de hemorragia intensa.

243. Hemorroides, almorranas - (em-oh-rroy-des, all-moh-rrah-nas)
Translation: Hemorrhoids
English: The doctor will be able to see the hemorrhoids through the scope.
Spanish: A través del anoscopio, el doctor será capaz de ver las hemorroides.

244. Hernia - (air-nee-ah)

Translation: Hernia

English: Though there are many causes of lower back pain, the culprit is often a herniated disc or arthritis.

Spanish: Aunque son muchas las causas del dolor lumbar, la responsable con frecuencia es una hernia de disco o artritis.

245. Hipo - (ee-poh)

Translation: Hiccups

English: Hiccups are common and normal in newborns and infants.

Spanish: El hipo es común y normal en recién nacidos y en bebés.

DAY 24

246. Zumbido en los o dos (zoom-bee-doh en los oh-EE-dohs)
Translation: Ringing in the ears
English: Very high doses of aspirin can increase risk for temporary hearing loss or ringing in the ear.
Spanish: Dosis muy altas de aspirina pueden incrementar el riesgo de pérdida auditiva temporal o zumbido en los oídos.

247. Ronquera (rron-kare-ah)
Translation: Hoarseness
English: A physical examination can determine whether hoarseness is caused by a respiratory tract infection.
Spanish: Un examen físico puede determinar si la ronquera es causada por una infección del tracto respiratorio.

248. Bochornos, calores, fogaje, sofocones - (boh-chor-nos, kah-lor-es)
Translation: Hot flashes
English: These drugs will produce symptoms of menopause like hot flashes and night sweats, in many women.
Spanish: Estos medicamentos producirán síntomas de menopausia como bochornos, sudoraciones nocturnas, en muchas mujeres.

249. Hipertensi n, tensi n alta (ee-pare-ten-see-YOHN)
Translation: Hypertension/high blood pressure
English: If untreated, severe hypertension may cause dangerous seizures and even death in the mother and fetus.
Spanish: Si no se trata, la hipertensión grave puede causar convulsiones peligrosas e incluso la muerte de la madre y del feto.

250. Histeria - (ees-tare-ee-ah)

Translation: Hysteria

English: Today, cases of hysteria have virtually disappeared.

Spanish: Hoy en día los casos de histeria son prácticamente inexistentes.

251. Enfermo, malo - (en-fare-moh/mah)

Translation: ill, sick

English: I was sick yesterday and could not attend the meeting.

Spanish: Ayer estuve enfermo y no pude asistir a la reunión.

252. Incontinencia, "no puede aguantar", "angurria" - (en-kon-tee-nen-see-yah)

Translation: Incontinence

English: Your bladder experiences a decline in its capacity and its tissues disintegrate causing incontinence.

Spanish: La vejiga experimenta una disminución en su capacidad y sus tejidos se desintegran causando incontinencia.

253. Indigesti n, "empacho" - (en-dee-hest-ee-YOHN)

Translation: Indigestion

English: This causes pain, indigestion and sometimes bleeding.

Spanish: Éstas provocan dolor, indigestión y, en ocasiones, hemorragia.

254. Infecci n, "enconarse" - (en-feck-SYOHN)

Translation: Infection

English: Infection can be treated with drainage and antibiotics, but will prolong your hospital stay.

Spanish: La infección puede ser tratada con drenajes y antibióticos, pero prolongará su permanencia en el hospital.

255. Inflamaci n, hinchaz n - (en-flah-mah-SYOHN)
Translation: Inflammation, swelling
English: Hepatitis is an inflammation, or swelling, of the liver.
Spanish: La hepatitis es una inflamación, o hinchazón, del hígado.

DAY 25

256. U a encarnada/enterrada, u ero (oon-yah en-kar-nah-dah/en-teh-rrah-dah)
Translation: Ingrown nail
English: If your toenail is very ingrown, your doctor might suggest minor surgery to remove all or part of the ingrown nail.
Spanish: Si la uña está muy encarnada, es posible que su médico sugiera la idea de una cirugía menor para retirar toda o parte de la uña encarnada.

257. Demencia, demente, loco (deh-men-see-ah, deh-men-tay)
Translation: Dementia, insanity, insane
English: Extra costs associated with old age are above all related to heart disease and cancer, followed by dementia.
Spanish: En cuanto a los ancianos, los costos extraordinarios provienen de enfermedades cardíacas y cáncer, seguidos por la demencia.

258. Insensibilidad, "que no siente" - (en-sens-ee-beel-ee-dahd)
Translation: Insensibility, numbness
English: If small nerve damage occurs, this can cause the patient to experience numbness in the lower lip and chin.
Spanish: Si se produce un daño en los nervios pequeños, esto puede causar que el paciente experimente insensibilidad en el labio inferior y en el mentón.

259. Insomnio, "no puede dormir" (en-som-nee-oh)
Translation: Insomnia
English: A dose taken too late in the day will cause insomnia.
Spanish: Una dosis tomada muy tarde en el día causará insomnio.

260. Pulso irregular - (pool-soh ee-rreg-oo-lahr)
Translation: Irregular pulse
English: An irregular pulse can also indicate a problem.

Spanish: Un pulso irregular también puede indicar un problema.

261. Irritaci n - (ee-rree-tah-SYOHN)
Translation: Irritation
English: Does your skin sometimes feel dry or irritated after shaving?
Spanish: ¿Siente irritación o sequedad en la piel después del afeitado?

262. Comez n, picaz n, escosor, "picor", "rasquera", "rasqui a", rascaz n" - (koh-may-SOHN)
Translation: Itch
English: Eczema causes the skin to itch, turn red, and flake.
Spanish: El eczema provoca comezón, enrojecimiento y escamación.

263. Ictericia, "piel amarillenta" - (ick-tare-ee-see-ah)
Translation: Jaundice
English: If your baby appears to be jaundiced, notify your pediatrician.
Spanish: Si su bebé parece tener ictericia, hay que notificar al pediatra.

264. Falta de apetito, no siente hambre - (fahl-tah day ah-pay-tee-toh)
Translation: Lack of appetite
English: If poor appetite and weight loss persist, discuss possible medicinal management with the patient's healthcare team.
Spanish: Si la falta de apetito y la pérdida de peso persisten, analice con el médico del paciente la posibilidad de empezar un tratamiento a base de medicamentos.

265. Cojera - (koh-hare-ah)

Translation: Limp/limping

English: If your child is limping, contact your pediatrician promptly for an evaluation.

Spanish: Si su hijo tiene cojera, contacte a su pediatra oportunamente para que le practique una evaluación.

DAY 26

SIGNS & SYMPTOMS - SEÑALES Y SÍNTOMAS

266. Laringitis (lahr-een-hee-tis)
Translation: Laryngitis
English: Your child, because of the current symptoms, has been diagnosed with laryngitis.
Spanish: Su hijo, por los síntomas que presenta en este momento, ha sido diagnosticado de laringitis.

267. Lesi n (Leh-SYOHN)
Translation: Lesion/injury
English: Has there been any recent history of an accident or injury?
Spanish: ¿Ha habido algún antecedente reciente de accidente o lesión?

268. Letargo, desgano, decaimiento - (leh-tar-goh)
Translation: Lethargy/lethargic
English: Increased production of melatonin can cause sleepiness and lethargy.
Spanish: El aumento de la producción de melatonina puede causar somnolencia y letargo.

269. Ceceo (seh-say-oh)
Translation: Lisp
English: My six year old has a frontal lisp when pronouncing words with S or Z.
Spanish: Mi hijo de seis años ha desarrollado un ceceo con las palabras que comienzan con S o Z.

270. Mand bula cerrada/desencajada - (mahn-DEE-boo-lah seh-rrah-dah, des-en-kah-hah-dah)

Translation: Locked jaw

English: Such spasms lead to lockjaw, which prevents opening or closing of the mouth.

Spanish: Estos espasmos ocasionan un trismo (mandíbula cerrada), que impide abrir o cerrar la boca.

271. Rodilla bloqueada - (roh-dee-yah bloh-kay-ah-dah)

Translation: Locked knee

English: If your knee locks up and is painful, your physician may determine that surgery is necessary to remove the damaged meniscus.

Spanish: Si su rodilla se bloquea y esto es doloroso, su médico puede determinar qué cirugía es necesaria para sacar el menisco dañado.

272. Dientes flojos - (dee-en-tes flo-hos)

Translation: Loose teeth

English: Do you have any loose teeth?

Spanish: ¿Tiene dientes flojos?

273. P rdida de - (PARE-dee-dah day)
Translation: Loss of

- appetite	- apetito
- balance	- equilibrio
- consciousness	- conocimiento
- coordination	- coordinación
- hair	- cabello/pelo
- memory	- memoria
- sexual desire	- deseo sexual
- voice	- voz

English: The main symptom is frequent, ongoing memory loss beyond what is normally expected for one's age.

Spanish: El síntoma principal es la pérdida de memoria de forma regular y constante que supera los niveles previstos para la edad de la persona.

274. Bajo peso al nacer - (bah-ho pay-soh al nah-sare)
Translation: Low birth weight

English: Women who are underweight may have babies with low birthweight.

Spanish: Las mujeres que se encuentran por debajo del peso normal pueden tener bebés con bajo peso al nacer.

275. Desnutrici n - (des-nu-tris-SYON)
Translation: Malnutrition

English: Hunger and malnutrition are common in many parts of the world.

Spanish: El hambre y la desnutrición son comunes en muchas partes del mundo.

DAY 27

276. Menopausia (meh-noh-pau-see-ah)

Translation: Menopause

English: Excessive sweating may also be a symptom of menopause.

Spanish: La sudoración excesiva también puede ser un síntoma de menopausia.

277. Flujo menstrual, "desecho" (flu-ho men-stroo-ahl)

Translation: Menstrual flow

English: Most of the menstrual fluid is extra tissue from the lining of the womb.

Spanish: La mayor parte del flujo menstrual es tejido excedente del revestimiento del útero.

278. Deterioro de la habilidad mental - (deh-tare-ee-or-oh day la ah-bee-lee-dahd men-tahl)

Translation: Mental ability impairment

English: It is used as a treatment for memory loss and mental impairment.

Spanish: Se utiliza como un tratamiento para la pérdida de memoria y el deterioro mental.

279. Migra a, jaqueca, dolor fuerte de cabeza (mee-grahn-yah)

Translation: Migraine

English: Getting too much or too little sleep, or napping during the day can trigger a migraine.

Spanish: Dormir demasiado o muy poco, o tomar siestas durante el día puede provocar una migraña.

280. Piel h meda - (pee-ehl oo-may-dah)
Translation: Damp/moist skin
English: Apply to damp skin, gently massage in and leave on for a moment.
Spanish: Aplicar sobre la piel húmeda, masajear suavemente y dejar actuar por un momento.

281. Lunar - (lu-nar)
Translation: Mole
English: I have a small mole on my nose.
Spanish: Tengo un pequeño lunar en la nariz.

282. Falta de coordinaci n, incoordinaci n muscular - (fahl-tah day koo-or-dee-nah-SYOHN)
Translation: Muscular incoordination
English: Strabismus is caused by a lack of coordination between the muscles in the eyes.
Spanish: El estrabismo es causado por una falta de coordinación entre los músculos de los ojos.

283. N usea, mareo "est mago revuelto" - (NOW-say-ah)
Translation: Nausea
English: Using a motion sickness wrist band may help control nausea.
Spanish: El uso de una pulsera contra mareos puede ayudar a controlar la náusea.

284. Sangrar por la nariz, hemorragia nasal - (sahn-grahr por la nah-rees)
Translation: Nose bleeding
English: Nose bleeding often can be controlled through direct pressure by pinching the nostrils with the fingers while sitting up.
Spanish: La hemorragia nasal severa se puede controlar con frecuencia aplicando presión directa y apretando las fosas nasales con los dedos y sentándose.

285. Entumecimiento, adormecimiento - (en-tu-mes-ee-mee-en-toh)

Translation: Numbness

English: Your doctor should identify and treat the underlying cause of your numbness or tingling.

Spanish: El médico debe identificar la causa subyacente del entumecimiento u hormigueo y luego tratarla.

DAY 28

286. Obstrucci n, "taponamiento" (ob-struk-SYOHN)
Translation: Blockage/obstruction
English: People who have a blockage of the intestines may need to avoid raw fruits and vegetables.
Spanish: Es posible que las personas que presenten obstrucción intestinal tengan que evitar las frutas y verduras crudas.

287. Dolor (doh-lohr)
Translation: Pain

- Dull   - sordo
- fulminant   - fulminante
- gripping   - opresivo
- Intense   - intenso, agudo
- irradiating   - que se irradia, que se corre
- persistent   - persistente, continuo, constante
- severe   - severo, muy fuerte

English: This is a common painkiller used for mild to moderate pain.
Spanish: Éste es un analgésico común usado para el dolor leve a moderado.

288. Enc as dolorosas - (en-SEE-ahs doh-loh-roh-sas)
Translation: Painful gums
English: You should also alert the doctor if you experience gum bleeding while pregnant.
Spanish: También le debería aconsejar al médico si experimenta sangrado de las encías durante el embarazo.

289. Palidez (pah-lee-des)

Translation: Paleness, pallor

English: The child may also experience sweating, nausea, or become pale.

Spanish: El niño puede experimentar sudores, náuseas o palidez.

290. Palpitaciones - (pahl-pee-tah-SYOHN-es)

Translation: Palpitations

English: Did you experience chest pain or heart palpitations when you fainted?

Spanish: ¿Experimentó dolor en el pecho o palpitaciones cardíacas cuando se desmayó?

291. Peladura, descamaci n de la piel - (peh-lah-doo-rah)

Translation: Skin peeling

English: Skin peeling on sunburned areas several days after the sunburn is normal.

Spanish: Peladura de la piel en áreas quemadas por el sol varios días después de la quemadura solar es normal.

292. Cosquilleo, hormigueo - (kos-kee-yay-oh)

Translation: Tingling

English: Symptoms are a burning or tingling sensation and cramping in the front of your foot.

Spanish: Los síntomas son una sensación de ardor o cosquilleo y calambres en la parte delantera de su pie.

293. Pleures a - (plu-eh-SEE-ah)

Translation: Pleurisy

English: Early treatment of bacterial respiratory infections can prevent pleurisy.

Spanish: El tratamiento oportuno de las infecciones respiratorias bacterianas puede prevenir la pleuresía.

294. Pulmon a - (pool-moh-NEE-ah)

Translation: Pneumonia

English: You also should be vaccinated against hepatitis B, influenza, and pneumonia if you are not immune to these diseases.

Spanish: También debe recibir la vacuna contra la hepatitis B, la influenza (gripe) y la pulmonía si no es inmune a estas enfermedades.

295. P lipo - (POH-lee-poh)

Translation: Polyp

English: Depending on the size of the polyp, it may be removed.

Spanish: Dependiendo del tamaño del pólipo, se puede extirpar.

DAY 29

SIGNS & SYMPTOMS - SEÑALES Y SÍNTOMAS

296. Envejecimiento prematuro (en-vey-hes-ee-mee-en-toh pray-mah-too-roh)
Translation: Premature aging
English: In the long term, it could increase the risk of skin and eye cancer, and cause the skin to age prematurely.
Spanish: A largo plazo, podrían aumentar el riesgo de padecer cáncer de piel y cáncer ocular, así como provocar el envejecimiento prematuro de la piel.

297. Eyaculaci n prematura/r pida, "venirse antes" (ee-yahk-oo-lah-SYOHN prey-mah-too-rah/RAH-pee-dah)
Translation: Premature ejaculation
English: Calcium channel blockers may help reduce premature ejaculation.
Spanish: Los bloqueadores del canal de calcio podrían ayudar a reducir la eyaculación prematura.

298. Menopausia prematura - (men-oh-paws-ee-ah prey-mah-too-rah)
Translation: Premature menopause
English: When menopause occurs before the age of 40 it is called premature menopause.
Spanish: Cuando la menopausia llega antes de los 40 años se le denomina menopausia prematura.

299. S ndrome premestrual (SEEN-droh-may prey-men-stroo-ahl)
Translation: Premenstrual syndrome (PMS)
English: Premenstrual syndrome (PMS) is the physical and psychological changes that occur before menstruation.
Spanish: El síndrome premenstrual (SPM) son los cambios físicos y psíquicos que se producen antes de la menstruación.

300. Prolapso del tero, "ca da de la matriz" - (pro-lap-soh del OO-tare-oh)
Translation: Uterine prolapse
English: Uterine prolapse occurs when the uterus slips out of place and into the vaginal canal due to weakening of the muscles and ligaments of the lower abdomen.
Spanish: El prolapso uterino se produce cuando el útero se desprende y cae sobre el canal vaginal debido al debilitamiento de los músculos y los ligamentos de la parte inferior del abdomen.

301. Postraci n, debilidad, abatimiento - (pos-trah-SYOHN)
Translation: Postration, weakness
English: Symptoms of heatstroke and heat prostration include: headache, dizziness, nausea or abdominal discomfort, rapid increase or decrease in pulse rate, and fainting or unconsciousness.
Spanish: Los síntomas de insolación y postración por calor incluyen: dolor de cabeza, mareo, nausea o malestar estomacal, aumento o disminución rápida del pulso y desmayo o pérdida del conocimiento.

302. Hinchaz n, intumescencia, abogotamiento - (een-cha-SOHN)
Translation: Puffiness
English: If you wake to puffy eyes, splash your face with cool water to help reduce the appearance of puffiness.
Spanish: Si se despierta con los ojos hinchados lave su cara con agua fresca para reducir la hinchazón.

303. Salpullido, sarpullido, erupci n, urticaria - (sahl-pool-ee-doh)

Translation: Rash

English: Stop using this medication and call your doctor if you have a rash.

Spanish: Pare de usar está medicina y llame a su médico si usted tiene un salpullido.

304. Reca da - (rey-kye-EE-dah)

Translation: Relapse/recurrence

English: We need to determine why this is occurring, so we can develop therapies to prevent it or prevent recurrence.

Spanish: Tenemos que determinar lo que ocurre, para que podamos desarrollar terapias preventivas o prevenir la recaída.

305. Intranquilidad - (en-trahn-kee-lee-dahd)

Translation: Restlessness

English: Besides pain, many people experience restlessness and agitation after surgery.

Spanish: Además del dolor, muchas personas experimentan inquietud y perturbación después de la cirugía.

DAY 30

SIGNS & SYMPTOMS - SEÑALES Y SÍNTOMAS

306. Fiebre reum tica (fee-ay-bray roo-MAH-tee-kah)
Translation: Rheumatic fever
English: Rheumatic fever is a rare complication of throat infection, that can damage the heart.
Spanish: La fiebre reumática es una complicación rara de la faringitis, que puede ocasionar daños en el corazón.

307. Reumatismo, "reuma", "riuma" (ray-oom-ah-tees-moh)
Translation: Rheumatism
English: Hemp fabric is ideal for sensitive skin and for people suffering from rheumatism.
Spanish: la tela de cáñamo es ideal para pieles sensibles y para las personas que sufren de reumatismo.

308. Cicatriz, marca - (sik-ah-treez, mar-kah)
Translation: Scar
English: Keep in mind that it is normal for a scar to form.
Spanish: Tenga en cuenta que es normal que se forme una cicatriz.

309. Rasgu o, raspadura (rahs-goon-yoh)
Translation: Scratch
English: Many times a child's injury will be no more severe than a bump, bruise or scratch.
Spanish: Muchas veces la lesión del niño no será más grave que un golpe, un moretón o un rasguño.

310. Ataques, convulsiones, episodios - (ah-tah-kays, kon-vool-see-ohn-es)

Translation: Convulsions, seizures

English: Seizures may be due to neurological problems and require further medical follow up.

Spanish: Las convulsiones pueden deberse a problemas neurológicos y requieren seguimiento médico.

311. T mido, vergonzoso - (TEEM-ee-doh/dah, ver-gon-zoh-soh/sah)

Translation: Shy

English: There are no precise guidelines for when a family should seek professional assistance for a shy child.

Spanish: No existen pautas precisas sobre cuándo la familia debería buscar ayuda profesional para un niño tímido.

312. Se al - (sen-yahl)

Translation: Sign

English: This is a common sign and symptom of sickle disease.

Spanish: Ésta es una señal y síntoma común de la anemia drepanocítica.

313. Cambio de color de la piel - (kam-bee-yoh day koh-lohr day la pee-ehl)

Translation: Skin discoloration

English: A dermatologist may also be able to recommend medications to help reduce skin darkening or discoloration.

Spanish: Un dermatólogo también podrá recomendarle medicamentos que disminuyan el oscurecimiento o el cambio de color de la piel.

314. Estornudo, estornudar - (es-tor-noo-doh)

Translation: Sneeze

English: The doctor will watch to see if you have an allergic reaction, such as sneezing or trouble breathing.

Spanish: El médico observará si tiene una reacción alérgica, por ejemplo, estornudo o dificultad al respirar.

315. Ronquido, roncar - (ron-kee-doh)

Translation: Snore

English: The smaller the airway, the more obstruction, and the louder the snoring.

Spanish: Mientras más reducida se encuentre la vía, mayor será la obstrucción y más fuerte el ronquido.

DAY 31

316. Llaga, lcera (yah-gah, OOL-sare-ah)
Translation: Sore, ulcer
English: When the ulcer is in the stomach, it is called a gastric ulcer.
Spanish: Cuando la úlcera está en el estómago, se llama úlcera gástrica.

317. Dolor de garganta (doh-lohr day la gar-gahn-tah)
Translation: Sore throat
English: You may also feel sick to your stomach, and have a dry mouth, sore throat, or feel cold or restless until the anesthesia wears off.
Spanish: También puede sentir náuseas, tener la boca reseca, dolor de garganta, o sentir frío o inquietud hasta que el efecto de la anestesia pase.

318. Espasmo - (es-pahs-moh)
Translation: Spasm, twitching
English: After you get treated, your health care provider should look for the cause of the spasm so that it doesn't recur.
Spanish: Después de recibir tratamiento, el médico debe buscar la causa del espasmo para evitar que se vuelva a presentar.

319. Espasticidad (es-pahs-tis-ee-dahd)
Translation: Spasticity
English: Most children with cerebral palsy have spasticity.
Spanish: La mayoría de los niños que sufren de parálisis cerebral tienen espasticidad.

320. Trastornos del habla, problemas para hablar - (Trahs-tor-nohs del ah-blah)

Translation: Speech difficulties

English: A speech pathologist specializes in speech and language disorders.

Spanish: Un patólogo del habla es especialista en trastornos del habla y lenguaje.

321. U as partidas/quebradizas - (oon-yahs par-tee-dahs/kay-brah-dees-ahs)

Translation: Split nails

English: Use moisturizer to help prevent dryness, splitting, and hangnails.

Spanish: Utilice un humectante para prevenir la resequedad, uñas partidas, y piel levantada conocida como padrastro.

322. Esguince, torcedura - (tor-say-doo-rah)

Translation: Sprain

English: A sprain is a partial or complete tear of a ligament.

Spanish: Un esguince es un desgarro parcial o completo de un ligamento.

323. Cuello r gido, "pescuezo tiezo" - (kway-yoh REE-hee-doh)

Translation: Stiff neck

English: Your child's neck is stiff.

Spanish: El cuello de su hijo está rígido.

324. Tartamudeo - (tar-tah-moo-day-oh)

Translation: Stuttering

English: Stuttering usually begins between the second and fourth birthday.

Spanish: El tartamudeo comienza por lo general entre 2 y 4 años de edad.

325. Dificultad al pasar/tragar - (dif-ee-kool-tahd ahl pah-sar / trah-gar)
Translation: Difficulty swallowing
English: If the cancer is large enough, it may cause difficulty swallowing.
Spanish: Si el cáncer es lo suficientemente grande, puede causar dificultad al tragar.

DAY 32

326. Trombosis (trom-boh-sis)
Translation: Thrombosis
English: Dehydration is the most common cause of renal vein thrombosis in infants.
Spanish: La deshidratación es la causa más común de trombosis de la vena renal en bebés.

327. Dolor de muela (doh-lohr day mway-lah)
Translation: Toothache
English: Most toothaches are a result of a cavity.
Spanish: La mayoría de los dolores de muela son originados por caries.

328. Ligamento roto, desgarramiento, esguince - (lig-ah-men-toh roh-toh)
Translation: Torn ligament
English: Sometimes, surgery to repair a torn ligament is needed.
Spanish: Algunas veces, se necesita cirugía para reparar un ligamento roto.

329. Temblor (tem-blore)
Translation: Tremor
English: Does the tremor impair your ability to use your hands or other body parts?
Spanish: ¿Altera el temblor la capacidad para usar las manos u otras partes del cuerpo?

330. Tumor - (too-more)

Translation: Tumor

English: Symptoms vary depending on the size and location of tumor.

Spanish: Los síntomas varían dependiendo del tamaño y la ubicación del tumor.

331. Sacudida nerviosa, "tic nervioso" - (sah-koo-dee-dah nare-vee-oh-sah)

Translation: Twitch, nervous tic

English: He used to save the shavings from his pencils that, out of nervous habit, he whittled down to the eraser.

Spanish: Guardaba las virutas de sus lápices que, debido a un tic nervioso, afilaba hasta la goma.

332. P rdida del conocimiento - (PARE-dee-dah del koh-nohs-ee-mee-en-toh)

Translation: Unconsciousness

English: A longer, deeper state of unconsciousness is often called a coma.

Spanish: El estado de pérdida del conocimiento más prolongado y más profundo a menudo se denomina coma.

333. Urticaria, "engranamiento" - (oor-tee-kar-ee-ah)

Translation: Urticaria, hives

English: Occasionally, a patient will develop itching and hives.

Spanish: En forma ocasional, un paciente desarrollará comezón y urticaria.

334. Venas varicosas, v rices - (vay-nahs bar-ee-koh-sahs)
Translation: Varicose veins
English: Treatment time is about 20 minutes but may be longer or shorter depending on the severity of the veins.
Spanish: El tratamiento requiere unos 20 minutos, aunque puede ser más prolongado o más corto, según la gravedad de las venas varicosas.

335. V rtigo, vahido - (BARE-tee-goh)
Translation: Dizziness
English: How would you describe the dizziness that you felt before fainting?
Spanish: ¿Cómo describiría el vértigo que sintió antes de desmayarse?

DAY 33

SIGNS & SYMPTOMS - SEÑALES Y SÍNTOMAS

336. V mito, "volver/deponer del est mago" (VOH-mee-toh)
Translation: Vomit
English: You may be asked to provide a sample of the stool or vomit for testing.
Spanish: Puede ser que le tomen una muestra de heces o vómito para examinarlas.

337. Verruga (bare-rroo-gah)
Translation: Wart
English: The typical wart is a raised round or oval growth on the skin with a rough surface.
Spanish: La verruga típica es un crecimiento redondo u oval con una superficie áspera.

338. Ojos llorosos - (oh-hos yor-oh-sos)
Translation: Watery eyes
English: More women than men say they suffer from seasonal eye allergies that lead to itchy, watery eyes.
Spanish: Más mujeres que hombres dicen sufrir alergias oculares estacionales que les causan irritación y ojos llorosos.

339. Respiraci n sibilante/silbante/"con pitido" (res-peer-ah-SYOHN sib-ee-lahn-tay)
Translation: Wheezing
English: Wheezing may be more common in viral pneumonia.
Spanish: La respiración sibilante es más frecuente en la neumonía vírica.

340. Arrugas - (ah-rroo-gahs)
Translation: Wrinkles
English: It helps reduce wrinkle formation.
Spanish: Ayuda a reducir la formación de arrugas.

341. Bostezo, bostezar - (bohs-tay-zoh, bohs-tay-zar)
Translation: Yawn
English: Is the yawning the same throughout the day?
Spanish: ¿Es el bostezo igual durante todo el día?

342. Orzuelo, "perrilla" - (or-zway-loh)
Translation: Stye, hordeolum
English: The initial symptom is a small swelling on the eyelid that often looks like a stye.
Spanish: El síntoma inicial es una pequeña inflamación en el párpado que, en ocasiones, se ve como un orzuelo.

343. Laga a, "chingui a" - (lah-gahn-yah)
Translation: Rheum, discharge (eyes)
English: There is red eye, with or without discharge.
Spanish: Uno de los ojos está enrojecido, con o sin lagañas.

344. Escorbuto - (es-kor-boo-toh)
Translation: Scurvy
English: Scurvy is a condition caused by an insufficient amount of vitamin C for a prolonged period of time.
Spanish: El escorbuto es una condición provocada por una cantidad insuficiente de vitamina C durante un período prolongado.

345. Piorrea - (pee-oh-rray-ah)
Translation: Pyorrhea, gum disease
English: This can result in tooth decay, worsen gum disease, and lead to tooth loss.
Spanish: Esto puede derivar en caries, empeoramiento de la piorrea y pérdida de dientes.

DAY 34

MEDICAL EXAMINATION - EXAMEN MÉDICO

346. Nombre (nohm-bray)
Translation: Name
English: What is your name?
Spanish: ¿Cuál es su nombre?

347. Apellido (ah-pay-yee-doh)
Translation: Last name
English: What is your last name?
Spanish: ¿Cuál es su apellido

348. Direcci n, domicilio - (dee-rek-SYOHN)
Translation: Address
English: What is your address?
Spanish: ¿Cuál es su dirección?

349. Direcci n/domicilio permanente (dee-rek-SYOHN pare-mah-nen-tay)
Translation: Permanent address
English: What is your permanent address?
Spanish: ¿Cuál es su dirección permanente?

350. Tel fono - (teh-LAY-foh-noh)
Translation: Telephone
English: I use the telephone to communicate with my clients.
Spanish: Uso el teléfono para comunicarme con mis clientes.

351. Fecha de nacimiento - (fay-cha day nah-see-mee-en-toh)
Translation: Date of birth
English: Complete the form with your name and date of birth.
Spanish: Rellene el formulario son su nombre y fecha de nacimiento.

352. Estatura, altura - (es-tah-too-rah, ahl-too-rah)

Translation: Height

English: I'm not sure of his exact height but he looks really tall.

Spanish: No sé cuál es su estatura exacta pero se ve muy alto.

353. Peso - (pay-soh)

Translation: Weight

English: How much do you weigh?

Spanish: ¿Cuál es su peso?

354. Grupo tnico, raza - (gru-poh ET-nee-koh)

Translation: Ethnic group

English: No ethnicity or race is more likely to have the condition.

Spanish: Sin embargo, ningún grupo étnico o raza era más propenso a tener la condición.

355. N mero de seguro social - (NU-mare-oh dy seh-goo-roh soh-see-ahl)

Translation: Social security number

English: You will be asked to provide the last four digits of your social security number for validation purposes.

Spanish: Se le pedirá que proporcione los últimos cuatro dígitos de su número de seguro social para fines de validación.

DAY 35

MEDICAL EXAMINATION - EXAMEN MÉDICO

356. Seguro m dico, "aseguranza" (seh-goo-roh MEH-dee-koh)
Translation: Medical/health insurance
English: Thankfully, half of the residents had health care.
Spanish: Afortunadamente, la mitad de los residentes tenían seguro médico.

357. P liza (POH-lee-zah)
Translation: Policy
English: The insurance policy covers all liabilities.
Spanish: La póliza de seguros cubre todas las responsabilidades.

358. Estado civil - (es-tah-doh see-vill)
Translation: Marital status

- married	- casado(a)
- single	- soltero(a)
- divorced	- divorciado(a)
- widower	- viudo
- widow	- viuda
- living together	- unión libre

English: You need to indicate your marital status in the form.
Spanish: Necesita indicar su estado civil en el formulario.

359. Contacto en caso de emergencia (kon-tahk-toh en ka-soh day eh-mur-hen-see-ah)
Translation: Emergency contact
English: It is extremely important that you provide us with current emergency telephone numbers.
Spanish: Es extremadamente importante que tengamos sus números actuales de contacto en caso de emergencia.

360. Ocupaci n, trabajo - (ahk-oo-pah-SYOHN)
Translation: Occupation
English: What's your occupation?
Spanish: ¿Cuál es su ocupación?

361. Lugar de trabajo - (loo-gar day trah-ba-ho)
Translation: Place of work, workplace
English: All workers wear hard hats in the workplace.
Spanish: Todos los obreros llevan casco en el lugar de trabajo.

362. Nombre del empleador/empresa/patr n - (nohm-bray del em-play-ah-dor)
Translation: Employer's name
English: Give the surnames and forenames of the employer.
Spanish: Indicar los apellidos y el nombre del empleador.

363. Ingresos mensuales, cu nto gana por mes - (en-greh-sohs men-soo-ahl-es)
Translation: Monthly income
English: Thanks to my promotion, my monthly income has increased.
Spanish: Gracias a mi ascenso, mis ingresos mensuales han aumentado.

364. Lugar de nacimiento - (loo-gar day nas-ee-mee-en-toh)
Translation: Birthplace
English: Indicate your birthplace and birthdate on the form.
Spanish: Indique su lugar de nacimiento y su fecha de nacimiento en la planilla.

365. Tel fono del trabajo - (teh-LAY-foh-no del trah-bah-ho)

Translation: Work phone

English: Write your work telephone number and employer's name on the application.

Spanish: Escriba el número de teléfono del trabajo y el nombre de su empleador en la solicitud.

DAY 36

MEDICAL HISTORY - HISTORIA MÉDICA

366. Seguro m dico (seh-goo-roh MEH-dee-koh)
Translation: Medical/health insurance
English: Thankfully, half of the residents had health care.
Spanish: Afortunadamente, la mitad de los residentes tenían seguro médico.

367. P liza (POH-lee-zah)
Translation: Policy
English: The insurance policy covers all liabilities.
Spanish: La póliza de seguros cubre todas las responsabilidades.

368. Estado civil - (es-tah-doh see-vill)
Translation: Marital status
English: You need to indicate your marital status in the form.
Spanish: Necesita indicar su estado civil en el formulario.

369. Contacto en caso de emergencia (kon-tahk-toh en ka-soh day eh-mur-hen-see-ah)
Translation: Emergency contact
English: It is extremely important that you provide us with current emergency telephone numbers.
Spanish: Es extremadamente importante que tengamos sus números actuales de contacto en caso de emergencia.

370. ¿Usted fuma? - (ooh-sted foo-mah)
Translation:
English: Do you smoke?

371. ¿Usted bebe/toma licor/alcohol? - (oo-sted bay-bay/toh-mah lee-kor/al-kohl)
Translation:
English: Do you drink alcohol?

372. ¿Cu nto? - (nohm-bray del em-play-ah-dor)
Translation:
English: How much?

373. ¿Desde hace cu nto tiempo? - (des-day ah-say kwan-toh)
Translation:
English: For how long?

374. ¿Tiene alergias? - (tee-en-ay ah-LEHR-hee-ahs)
Translation:
English: Do you have allergies?

375. Medicinas o drogas que est usando actualmente
Translation:
English: Medicines or drugs you are using currently

DAY 37

HELPFUL PHRASES - FRASES ÚTILES

376. ¿Ha tenido alguna de las siguientes enfermedades?
Translation:
English: Have you ever had any of the following illnesses?

377. ¿Algún miembro de su familia ha tenido alguna de estas enfermedades?
Translation:
English: Has any member of your family had any of the following illnesses?

378. ¿Dónde ha vivido la mayor parte de su vida?
Translation:
English: Where have you lived for most of your life?

379. ¿Tiene usted alguno de estos síntomas?
Translation:
English: Do you have any of the following symptoms?

GENERAL INSTRUCTIONS - INSTRUCCIONES GENERALES

380. Desvístase por completo, quítese toda la ropa
Translation:
English: Take off all your clothes

381. Desvístase de la cintura para arriba/cintura para abajo
Translation:
English: Undress from the waist up/waist down.

382. P ngase esta bata
Translation:
English: Put on this gown

383. Si ntese sobre la mesa
Translation:
English: Sit on the table

384. Acu stese sobre la mesa
Translation:
English: Lie down on the table

385. Acu stese de medio lado
Translation:
English: Lie on your side

DAY 38

GENERAL INSTRUCTIONS - INSTRUCCIONES GENERALES

386. P ngase boca arriba
Translation:
English: Turn face up

387. P ngase boca abajo
Translation:
English: Turn face down

388. Rel jese, afloje/suelte el cuerpo
Translation:
English: Relax

389. Extienda/estire sus brazos
Translation:
English: Extend your arms

390. Doble las rodillas
Translation:
English: Bend your knees

391. Se ale/apunte donde le duele
Translation:
English: Point where you feel the pain

392. Avise/diga/indique cuando sienta dolor
Translation:
English: Say when you feel the pain

393. Mire hacia el frente
Translation:

English: Keep your eyes to the front

394. Abra la boca
Translation:
English: Open your mouth

395. Saque la lengua
Translation:
English: Stick your tongue out

DAY 39

GENERAL INSTRUCTIONS - INSTRUCCIONES GENERALES

396. Respire profundo/hondo
Translation:
English: Take a deep breath

397. Respire lento/despacio
Translation:
English: Breathe slowly

398. Respire rápido
Translation:
English: Breathe quickly

399. Aguante la respiración
Translation:
English: Hold your breath

400. Voy a:

Translation:

English: I am going to:

- take your pulse	- tomarle el pulso
- take your blood pressure	- tomarle la presión arterial/tensión
- measure you	- medirlo(a)
- weight you	- pesarlo(a)
- take a blood sample	- tomarle una muestra de sangre
- take a sputum sample	- tomarle una muestra de esputo/flema
- take some x-rays	- sacarle unos rayos equis/radiografías/placas
- give you an enema	- ponerle un enema/lavativa/lavado intestinal

401. Venga en ayunas

Translation:

English: Come with an empty stomach

402. Acumule y traiga la orina de las Itimas 24 horas

Translation:

English: Collect and bring your urine from the previous 24 hours

403. Venga con la vejiga llena

Translation:

English: Come with a full bladder

404. No se mueva

Translation:

English: Don't move

405. Camine despacio

Translation:

English: Walk slowly

DAY 40

INSTITUTIONS AND CLINICS - INSTITUCIONES Y CLÍNICAS

406. Guarder a infantil

Translation: Child nursery, day care center

English: The department also provides for the cost of nursery and day care services when indicated.

Spanish: El departamento también cubre los gastos de guardería infantil cuando así procede.

407. Cl nica

Translation: clinic

English: Tony has been asking to see you down in the Clinic.

Spanish: Tony pide verlo en la Clínica.

408. Consultorio dental, "dentister a"

Translation: dental office

English: This is a dental practice.

Spanish: Esto es un consultorio dental.

409. Departamento de servicios de salud

Translation: department of health services

English: A new hospital was opened by the Health Services Department in George Town in April 1999.

Spanish: En abril de 1999 el Departamento de Servicios de Salud abrió un nuevo hospital en George Town.

410. Dispensario

Translation: dispensary

English: The Well Women's Clinic and the Lifetime Health Plan are examples of initiatives based on wellness.

Spanish: El Dispensario de la Mujer en Buen Estado de Salud, y el Plan de Salud Durante Toda la Vida son ejemplos de iniciativas basadas en la buena salud.

411. Consultorio m dico

Translation: doctor's office

English: The procedure can be done under local anesthesia in a doctor's office.

Spanish: El procedimiento puede hacerse bajo anestesia local en un consultorio médico.

412. Centro de salud

Translation: health center

English: We should get him to the health centre.

Spanish: Tenemos que llevarlo al centro de salud.

413. Departamento de salud/salubridad

Translation: health department

English: The health department shut it down six months ago.

Spanish: El Departamento de salud lo cerró hace seis meses.

414. Hospital

Translation: hospital

English: Follow me, we'll talk as we head for the Hospital.

Spanish: Síguame. Hablaremos mientras vamos al hospital.

415. Clínica de inmunizaciones/vacunas

Translation: immunization clinic

English: A child's birth could also be recorded when it was brought to a health clinic for immunization.

Spanish: También se puede registrar el nacimiento de un niño cuando se le lleva a una clínica para su inmunización.

DAY 41

INSTITUTIONS AND CLINICS - INSTITUCIONES Y CLÍNICAS

416. Laboratorio (lah-bor-ah-tor-ee-oh)
Translation: laboratory
English: I'll have her body diverted to the lab and start the protocol.
Spanish: Haré desviar su cuerpo al Laboratorio e iniciar el protocolo.

417. Hospital para enfermos mentales, manicomio, "asilo de locos"
Translation: mental hospital
English: I think there's a mental hospital near here.
Spanish: Creo que hay un manicomio cerca.

418. Ancianato, asilo de ancianos, casa para personas de la tercera edad
Translation: nursing home
English: I don't want him to go back to that nursing home.
Spanish: No quiero que regrese a ese ancianato.

419. Cl nica de consulta externa
Translation: outpatient clinic
English: The procedure is so simple that you don't need to stay in hospital, you can have it done at an outpatient clinic.
Spanish: La operación es tan simple que ni siquiera debes ir al hospital, puedes hacértela en una clínica para pacientes externos.

420. Farmacia, botica, droguer a
Translation: pharmacy
English: Could you tell me where the nearest pharmacy is?
Spanish: ¿Puede decirme dónde queda la farmacia más cercana?

421. Centro de planificaci n familiar

Translation: planned parenthood center

English: Well, there is no harm in visiting the family planning center just to see what your options are.

Spanish: Bueno, a nadie le hace daño una visita al centro de planificación familiar sólo para ver qué opciones tiene.

422. Centro de control de envenenamiento

Translation: poison control center

English: If swallowed, please contact the Poison Control Center immediately.

Spanish: Si se ingiriese, por favor contacten inmediatamente con el Centro de Control de Envenenamiento.

423. Sanatorio

Translation: sanatorium

English: His grandfather was in the asylum here.

Spanish: Su abuelo estvo aquí en el Sanatorio.

424. Cl nica del ni o sano, cl nica para ex menes de rutina para ni os

Translation: well-baby clinic

English: Your baby's doctor will check for this reflex right after birth and during well-child visits.

Spanish: El pediatra verificará este reflejo inmediatamente después del nacimiento y durante las consultas del niño sano.

425. Morgue, anfiteatro, dep sito de cad veres

Translation: morgue

English: Just looking for some reference photos for a mortuary.

Spanish: Estoy buscando fotos de una morgue.

DAY 42

IN THE HOSPITAL - EN EL HOSPITAL

426. Ambulancia
Translation: ambulance
English: Get me an ambulance and a med examiner.
Spanish: Necesito un médico y una ambulancia.

427. Cama
Translation: bed
English: A bed like that would be good to have.
Spanish: Una cama así sería bueno tener.

428. Bac n de cama, bacinica, "c modo", cu a
Translation: bedpan
English: Rosa found it difficult to use a bedpan immediately after the operation.
Spanish: Cuando estaba recién operada le resultaba difícil a Rosa usar la bacinica.

429. Encamado(a), postrado en cama
Translation: bedridden patient
English: Encourage movement and deep breathing in anyone who is bedridden for long periods.
Spanish: Estimule el movimiento y las respiraciones profundas en alguien postrado en cama por períodos prolongados.

420. Frazada, manta, cobija
Translation: blanket, blankie
English: I had that same blankie when I was a baby.
Spanish: Yo tenía esa misma frazada cuando era un bebé.

421. Timbre

Translation: call bell, buzzer

English: Now, if you want anything, just press the buzzer.

Spanish: Si necesita algo, presione el timbre.

422. Convaleciente

Translation: convalescent, recovering

English: She's in a convalescent hospital in Paris.

Spanish: Ella está convaleciente en un hospital en París.

423. Sala de parto

Translation: delivery room

English: I'll be there, in the delivery room, holding your hand.

Spanish: Estaré contigo en la sala de parto, sujetando tu mano.

424. Dar de alta

Translation: To discharge, to release from the hospital

English: In a few days we'll discharge you.

Spanish: En unos días le vamos a dar de alta.

425. Urgencias, sala de emergencia

Translation: emergency room (ER)

English: I have been in the emergency room all night.

Spanish: He estado en la sala de emergencia toda la noche.

DAY 43

IN THE HOSPITAL - EN EL HOSPITAL

426. Hospitalizar, internar
Translation: hospitalization
English: The decision to hospitalize a person has to be taken by a specialized physician, and only after he has personally conducted an examination.
Spanish: La decisión de hospitalizar a una persona debe ser tomada por un médico especialista y únicamente después de haberla examinado personalmente.

427. Hospitalizado(a), internado(a)
Translation: hospitalized
English: He's been hospitalised because of his injuries.
Spanish: Ha sido hospitalizado debido a sus lesiones.

428. Cuidado intensivo, terapia intensiva
Translation: intensive care
English: With any luck, we'll have her out of the ICU tomorrow.
Spanish: Con suerte, mañana saldrá de Cuidados Intensivos.

429. Sala de maternidad, "sala de gineco"
Translation: maternity ward
English: I'm needed at the maternity ward.
Spanish: Me necesitan en la sala de maternidad.

430. Paciente
Translation: patient
English: Right now, the hospital is treating two hundred patients.
Spanish: En este momento, el hospital está tratando a doscientos pacientes.

431. Almohada, cojín

Translation: pillow

English: If you get yourself a feather pillow you'll sleep like a baby.

Spanish: Compra una almohada de plumas y vas a dormir como un bebé .

432. Sala de recuperación

Translation: recovery room

English: He said he's in a recovery room.

Spanish: Dijo que está en la sala de recuperación.

433. Sala de rehabilitación

Translation: rehabilitation room

English: There's a physical therapy room down there.

Spanish: Abajo hay una sala de rehabilitación.

434. Habitación, sala, cuarto

Translation: room

English: A classic room with an excellent atmosphere.

Spanish: Una habitación clásica de excelente atmósfera.

435. Camilla

Translation: Stretcher

English: Bob, call for a stretcher, please.

Spanish: Bob, pide una camilla, por favor.

DAY 44

IN THE HOSPITAL - EN EL HOSPITAL

436. Sala de operaciones, quir fano
Translation: operating room,
English: We have an operating room waiting for him.
Spanish: Tenemos una sala de operaciones esperandole.

437. Orinal, "pato"
Translation: urinal
English: There is only one urinal in the corner.
Spanish: Hay solamente un orinal en la esquina.

438. Horas de visita
Translation: visiting hours
English: Lady... visiting hours are over.
Spanish: Señora, las horas de visita ya pasaron.

439. Sala de espera, vest bulo
Translation: waiting room
English: She's in the waiting room trying to get some sleep.
Spanish: Está en la sala de espera, intentando dormir.

440. Sala
Translation: ward
English: This is Observation Room B. We need help, stat.
Spanish: Sala de observación B. Necesitamos ayuda, ya.

441. Silla de ruedas
Translation: wheel chair
English: Can I get a wheelchair down here, please?
Spanish: ¿Puede alguien traerme una silla de ruedas, por favor?

442. Sala de rayos X
Translation: x-ray room
English: They took him down for an X-ray.
Spanish: Lo llevaron a la sala de rayos X.

443. Sala de parto
Translation: delivery room
English: I ran off to the delivery room.
Spanish: Fui corriendo hacia la sala de parto.

PERSONNEL/STAFF - PERSONAL

444. Alergista
Translation: allergist
English: I just went to see the allergist.
Spanish: Recién fui a ver al alergista.

445. Anestesista, anestesi logo(a)
Translation: anesthetist, anesthesiologist
English: It looks like the anesthesiologist increased oxygenation towards the end of the procedure.
Spanish: Parece que el Anestesista aumentó la oxigenación hacia el final de la intervención.

DAY 45

446. Quiropráctico
Translation: chiropractor
English: I think this woman has need of a chiropractor.
Spanish: Creo que esta mujer necesita un quiropráctico.

447. Consejero(a)
Translation: counselor, consultant, adviser
English: Juan is one of the advisers or consultants for the business group.
Spanish: Juan es uno de los consejeros del grupo empresarial.

448. Dermatólogo(a)
Translation: dermatologist
English: I had a dermatologist check it out and all the materials are hypoallergenic.
Spanish: Lo ha revisado un dermatólogo y todos los materiales son hipoalérgicos.

449. Dietista
Translation: dietitian
English: Work with your doctor and a dietician or nutritionist on a regular basis to develop the best plan for you.
Spanish: Trabaje con su médico y con su dietista o nutricionista regularmente para desarrollar el mejor plan para usted.

450. M dico(a), doctor(a)

Translation: doctor, physician

English: She rightly thought that such a condition should be investigated by your physician.

Spanish: Pensó correctamente que esa enfermedad debía ser investigada por su médico.

451. Epidemi logo(a)

Translation: epidemiologist

English: Now, I'm an infectious disease epidemiologist by training.

Spanish: Ahora, por formación, soy epidemiólogo.

452. Ginec logo(a)

Translation: gynecologist

English: You know, you might want to look around for a new gynecologist.

Spanish: Ya sabes, tal vez quieras buscar otra ginecóloga.

453. Auxiliares de salud

Translation: health aides

English: These are trained medical aides located in the rural communities to provide basic maternal and child care services.

Spanish: Estos están dotados de auxiliares de salud calificados asignados a las comunidades rurales para prestar servicios básicos de atención maternoinfantil.

454. Educador(a) de salud

Translation: health educator

English: Apart from one educator, the project is entirely run by very young participants.

Spanish: Aparte de un educador, el proyecto está totalmente dirigido por participantes muy jóvenes.

455. Personal de laboratorio

Translation: lab personnel

English: If the competence is considered unsatisfactory, a re-training of the laboratory staff shall be undertaken as the minimal corrective measure.

Spanish: Si las competencias no se consideran satisfactorias, se procederá a formar de nuevo al personal de laboratorio, como medida correctora mínima.

DAY 46

PERSONNEL/STAFF – PERSONAL

456. Neum logo(a)
Translation: lung specialist, respiratory physician
English: I was called down to the ward by a respiratory physician to see him.
Spanish: Un neumólogo me llamó a la sala para verlo.

457. Partera, comadrona, matrona
Translation: midwife
English: The midwife is in there for natural childbirth.
Spanish: La partera está allí para asistir en el parto natural.

458. Naturista
Translation: naturopath
English: The naturalist movement is growing.
Spanish: El movimiento naturista está en auge.

459. Neurocirujano(a)
Translation: neurosurgeon
English: The neurosurgeon is going to come in and talk to you.
Spanish: El neurocirujano vendrá y hablará con ustedes.

460. Enfermera(o)
Translation: nurse
English: A nurse will be here with you in case you need anything.
Spanish: Una enfermera estará aquí con usted si necesita algo.

461. Auxiliar de enfermer a

Translation: nurse's aid

English: The hospital has a nursing school, which trains practical nurses.

Spanish: Hay una escuela de enfermería en el Hospital, donde se puede obtener el grado de enfermera auxiliar.

462. Supervisor(a)/jefe(a) de enfermer a

Translation: nursing supervisor

English: Check with the nursing supervisor.

Spanish: Hable con la supervisora de enfermería.

463. Nutricionista, nutri logo(a)

Translation: nutritionist

English: Your doctor, nurse, or dietitian will recommend a diet for you.

Spanish: El médico, la enfermera o el nutricionista le recomendarán una dieta.

464. Obstetra, toc logo(a)

Translation: obstetrician

English: She wants to come with me tomorrow to the OB/GYN.

Spanish: Quiere acompañarme a ver al obstetra mañana.

465. Onc logo(a)

Translation: oncologist

English: I saw an oncologist when I first found out.

Spanish: Fui a un oncólogo cuando me lo diagnosticaron.

DAY 47

466. Oftalm logo(a), oculista
Translation: ophthalmologist, oculist
English: The ophthalmologist you saw found no indication of retinopathy.
Spanish: El oftalmólogo que vio no encontró indicaciones de retinopatía.

467. Optometrista
Translation: optometrist
English: The optometrist said you have a stigmatism.
Spanish: El optometrista dijo que tiene astigmatismo.

468. Ortopedista
Translation: orthopedist
English: He'll need to see an orthopedist when he gets back.
Spanish: Debemos pedir cita con un ortopedista apenas vuelva.

469. Oste pata
Translation: osteopath
English: My osteopath says that it's bad for my spine.
Spanish: Mi osteópata dice que es malo para mi columna.

470. Param dico
Translation: paramedic
English: The paramedic saved the burn victim on the way to the hospital.
Spanish: El paramédico salvó a la víctima quemada camino al hospital.

471. Pat logo(a)
Translation: pathologist
English: The pathologist wanted you to see it straight away.
Spanish: El patólogo quería que lo viera enseguida.

472. Pediatra
Translation: pediatrician
English: Your son was checked out by a pediatrician.
Spanish: Un pediatra examinó a su hijo.

473. Farmac utico, farmacista, boticario, dependiente de farmacia
Translation: pharmacist
English: I'll ask the pharmacist what to do.
Spanish: Le preguntaré al farmacéutico qué hacer.

474. Pod logo(a), podiatra, callista
Translation: podiatrist, chiropodist
English: Are you a podiatrist?
Spanish: ¿Es usted una podóloga?

475. Psiquiatra
Translation: psychiatrist
English: I became a psychiatrist because I wanted to understand the illness.
Spanish: Me convertí en psiquiatra porque quería entender la enfermedad.

DAY 48

476. Psic logo(a)
Translation: psychologist
English: As a psychologist, I am fascinated by the origin and consequences of such kindness.
Spanish: Como psicólogo, me fascinan el origen y las consecuencias de semejante bondad.

477. Enfermero(a) de salud p blica
Translation: public health nurse
English: The public health nurse helped the old person get up from the bed.
Spanish: La enfermera de salud pública ayudó al anciano a levantarse de la cama.

478. Radi logo(a)
Translation: radiologist, radiographer
English: The radiographer would like us to do some more testing.
Spanish: Al radiólogo le gustaría hacer otro estudio.

479. Trabajador(a) social
Translation: social worker
English: We've got the social worker on his way.
Spanish: Tenemos al trabajador social en camino.

480. Especialista
Translation: specialist
English: At least until we can get you checked out, by a specialist.
Spanish: Al menos hasta que pueda verlo un especialista.

481. Cirujano

Translation: surgeon

English: He's the best ocular surgeon I know.

Spanish: Él es el mejor cirujano ocular que conozco.

482. Terapista, terap uta

Translation: therapist

English: I know a therapist who could really help you.

Spanish: Conozco a un terapista que podría ayudarlo.

483. Enfermera de piso/planta

Translation: ward nurse

English: There are no female nurses on this floor.

Spanish: No hay enfermeras en este piso.

DAY 49

TREATMENT PROCEDURES - PROCEDIMIENTOS CURATIVOS

484. Transfusi n de sangre
Translation: blood transfusion
English: She will die without this blood transfusion.
Spanish: Morirá sin esta transfusión de sangre.

485. Quimioterapia
Translation: chemotherapy
English: We'll begin the chemotherapy sessions as soon as possible.
Spanish: Empezaremos las sesiones de quimioterapia lo antes posible.

486. Limpiar
Translation: To clean
English: You have to learn how to clean everything.
Spanish: Tiene que aprender a limpiar todo.

487. Desinfectar
Translation: To disinfect
English: We have to sanitize this place.
Spanish: Tenemos que "desinfectar" este lugar.

488. Duchas, lavados
Translation: Showers
English: At the end of the hallway there are toilets and showers.
Spanish: Al final del pasillo hay baños y duchas.

489. Tomar bastantes l quidos

Translation: To drink lots of fluids

English: Drink plenty of fluids to help prevent infections.

Spanish: Tome bastante líquido para ayudar a prevenir infecciones.

490. Enema, lavativa

Translation: enema

English: The doctor ordered an enema for the patient before the procedure.

Spanish: El doctor ordenó un enema para el paciente antes de su cirugía.

491. Tratamiento hormonal

Translation: hormone treatment

English: Hormonal treatment is used to trigger the last phase of egg maturation.

Spanish: El tratamiento hormonal es usado para gatillar la última fase de la maduración de los huevos.

492. Inyecci n, "piquete"

Translation: injection, shot

English: I'll give you a shot to calm down.

Spanish: Le daré una inyección para calmarlo.

493. Intravenosa

Translation: intravenous (IV)

English: He hasn't finished his I.V. Antibiotics.

Spanish: Él no ha terminado sus antibióticos por vía intravenosa.

494. Radioterapia, radiaciones

Translation: radiotherapy

English: We'll follow it up with radiotherapy and perhaps chemotherapy, as well.

Spanish: Seguiremos con la radioterapia y quizás quimioterapia también.

495. Ba o de asiento/de tina

Translation: sitz bath

English: Soaking in a warm bath (sitz bath) can help relieve pain.

Spanish: Remojarse en un baño caliente (baño de asiento) puede ayudar a aliviar el dolor.

DAY 50

496. Vendar
Translation: to bandage
English: I could use it to dress/bandage the wound.
Spanish: Podría usarlo para vendar la herida.

497. Hospitalizarse, ir al hospital
Translation: to be hospitalized
English: Patients must be hospitalised at the beginning of treatment due to symptoms of disease and to ensure adequate monitoring.
Spanish: Debe hospitalizarse a los pacientes al principio del tratamiento debido a los síntomas de la enfermedad y para asegurar una monitorización adecuada.

498. Estar en cama
Translation: to be in bed
English: Everyone else should be in bed.
Spanish: Todos los demás deben estar en cama.

499. Poner el brazo en cabestrillo/honda
Translation: to place the arm in sling
English: I'm afraid you'll have to carry that arm in a sling for a week or so.
Spanish: Me temo que tendrá que llevar el brazo en cabestrillo durante una semana.

500. Enyesar, poner yeso
Translation: to put in a cast
English: We'll put your arm in a cast and bandage the broken ribs.
Spanish: Le vamos a enyesar el brazo y vendar las costillas rotas.

501. Consultar a un especialista

Translation: to see a specialist

English: I will continue to help, but you need to consult a specialist.

Spanish: Voy a seguir ayudándolo, pero es necesario consultar a un especialista.

502. Entablillar

Translation: to splint

English: I need to splint your leg, and you're not going to be able to put any weight on it.

Spanish: Necesito entablillar su pierna, y no va a poder poner ningún peso sobre ella.

503. Operaci n

Translation: operation

English: I'll monitor the surgery while he operates.

Spanish: Monitorizaré la cirugía mientras él opera.

504. Descanso

Translation: rest

English: You know what? I think this would be a good time for a break.

Spanish: ¿Sabes qué? Creo que es un buen momento para un descanso.

DAY 51

INSTRUMENTS AND MATERIALS - INSTRUMENTOS Y MATERIALES

505. Cinta adhesiva, tafet n, esparadrapo
Translation:
English: **adhesive tape**

506. Alcohol
Translation:
English: **alcohol**

507. Venda
Translation:
English: **bandage**

508. Cura, curita, parche curita
Translation:
English: **band aid**

509. Vendaje
Translation:
English: **bandage**

510. Aparato ortop dico
Translation:
English: **brace**

511. Yeso
Translation:
English: **cast**

512. Catéter, sonda
Translation:
English: catheter

513. Algodón
Translation:
English: cotton

514. Hisopo, "palito con algodón"
Translation:
English: cotton swab

515. Muletas
Translation:
English: crutches

DAY 52

INSTRUMENTS AND MATERIALS - INSTRUMENTOS Y MATERIALES

516. Audioscopio
Translation:
English: earscope

517. Electrocardiograma, "electro"
Translation:
English: electrocardiogram (EKG)

518. Almohadilla el ctrica
Translation:
English: heating pad

519. Bolsa de agua caliente
Translation:
English: hot water bottle

520. Compresas/lienzos/fumentos de agua caliente
Translation:
English: hot wet compress

521. Bolsa de hielo
Translation:
English: ice pack

522. Gasa
Translation:
English: gauze

523. Microscopio
Translation:
English: microscope

524. Porta-objetos para microscopios
Translation:
English: microscope slides

525. Aguja
Translation:
English: needle

526. Parche
Translation:
English: patch

DAY 53

INSTRUMENTS AND MATERIALS - INSTRUMENTOS Y MATERIALES

527. Caja de Petri
Translation:
English: **Petri dish**

528. B scula, pesa, balanza
Translation:
English: **scale**

529. Esp culo, espejo vaginal
Translation:
English: **speculum**

530. Bauman metro
Translation:
English: **sphygmomanometer**

531. Estetoscopio
Translation:
English: **stethoscope**

532. Jeringa, jeringuilla
Translation:
English: **syringe**

533. Term metro
Translation:
English: **thermometer:**
    - ear   - de oído

- oral   - oral
- rectal - rectal

534. Abate lengua, pisa lengua, paleta
Translation:
English: tongue depressor

535. Diapas n
Translation:
English: tuning fork

DAY 54

MEDICATIONS – MEDICAMENTOS

536. Acetaminofeno
Translation: acetaminophen
English: Acetaminophen is used to mitigate pain.
Spanish: El acetaminofeno se usa para mitigar el dolor.

537. Adrenalina
Translation: adrenaline
English: I love base jumping for the adrenaline rush I get.
Spanish: Me encanta hacer salto base por el subidón de adrenalina que me da.

538. Analg sico
Translation: analgesic, painkiller
English: The dentist prescribed me painkillers to relieve the pain of my wisdom tooth.
Spanish: El dentista me mandó analgésicos para aliviar el dolor de la muela del juicio.

539. Anti cido
Translation: antacid
English: Lorena took antacid tablets when she was pregnant.
Spanish: Lorena tomaba pastillas antiácidas cuando estaba embarazada.

540. Antibi tico
Translation: antibiotic
English: If you don't take the antibiotics you will never get better.
Spanish: Si no te tomas los antibióticos nunca mejorarás.

541. Anticonvulsivo, anticonvulsivante

Translation: anticonvulsant

English: Your doctor may need to consider giving you a different anticonvulsant.

Spanish: Su médico considerar darle otro anticonvulsivante.

542. Anticuagulante

Translation: anticoagulant

English: Treatment usually involves anticoagulant medication.

Spanish: El tratamiento normalmente involucra medicamentos anticoagulantes.

543. Antidepresivo

Translation: antidepressant

English: He was taking an antipsychotic drug and an antidepressant.

Spanish: Estaba tomando un antipsicótico y un antidepresivo.

544. Antidiarreico

Translation: antidiarrheal

English: Calcium carbonate? That's an anti-diarrheal, right?

Spanish: Carbonato de calcio, eso es un antidiarreico, ¿verdad?

545. Ant doto

Translation: antidote

English: I administered the antidote about sixty-six seconds after the venom was injected.

Spanish: Me inyecté el antídoto 66 segundos después del veneno.

DAY 55

MEDICATIONS – MEDICAMENTOS

546. Antiem tico
Translation: antiemetic
English: The use of an anti-emetic may be necessary.
Spanish: Puede ser necesario administrar un antiemético.

547. Antihistam nico
Translation: antihistamine
English: I'm waiting for an antihistamine to take effect.
Spanish: Estoy esperando a que surta efecto un antihistamínico.

548. Anti-inflamatorio
Translation: anti-inflammatory
English: It's non-steroidal anti-inflammatory injection used to treat pain.
Spanish: Es la inyección anti-inflamatorio no esteroideo utilizado para tratar el dolor.

549. Antis ptico
Translation: antiseptic
English: Mr. Smith and I never travel without a bottle of antiseptic.
Spanish: El Sr. Smith y yo nunca viajamos sin una botella de antiséptico.

550. Antitusivo, b quico

Translation: antitussive, cough suppressant

English: You may need a prescription cough suppressant, but let me listen to your lungs first.

Spanish: Es posible que necesite una receta antitusivo pero déjeme escuchar sus pulmones primero.

551. Aspirina

Translation: aspirin

English: I have to get some aspirin to help her.

Spanish: Tengo que conseguir una aspirina para ayudarla.

552. Atropina

Translation: atropine

English: We've given her morphine, and atropine.

Spanish: Le hemos dado morfina y atropina.

553. Bicarbonato

Translation: bicarbonate

English: We should put him on a bi-carb drip and send him back.

Spanish: Deberíamos ponerle un goteo de bicarbonato y enviarlo de regreso.

554. Bromuto

Translation: bromide

English: Water stains on his heels show traces of sodium bromide.

Spanish: Las manchas de agua en sus tacones muestran rastros de bromuto de sodio.

555. Broncodilatador

Translation: bronchodilator

English: You should be prescribing it because it's the best xanthine bronchodilator on the market.

Spanish: Debería estar recetándolo porque es el mejor broncodilatador xantina del mercado.

DAY 56

MEDICATIONS – MEDICAMENTOS

556. C psulas
Translation: capsules
English: The capsule should be swallowed with some water.
Spanish: Las cápsulas deben tragarse con agua.

557. Code na
Translation: codeine
English: It's an opiate, commonly known as codeine.
Spanish: Es un opiáceo, se conoce vulgarmente como codeína.

558. Cortisona
Translation: cortisone
English: One example is cortisone, which is used to treat arthritis and other inflammatory diseases.
Spanish: Un ejemplo es la cortisona, empleada para tratar la artritis y otras enfermedades inflamatorias.

559. Descongestionante
Translation: decongestant
English: A treatment with a soothing, decongesting and lenitive effect.
Spanish: Tratamiento con efecto calmante, descongestionante y lenitivo.

560. Diur tico
Translation: diuretic
English: A moment ago though, we gave her a diuretic.
Spanish: Aunque hace un momento, le hayamos dado un diurético.

561. Gotas para los o dos

Translation: ear drops

English: Hello...! we need your wonderful ear drops again for little Sarah.

Spanish: Hola...! Necesitamos sus maravillosas gotas para los oídos de nuevo para la pequeña Sara.

562. Estr geno

Translation: estrogen

English: You'll be getting a daily estrogen shot.

Spanish: Recibirás una inyección diaria de estrógeno.

563. Expectorante

Translation: expectorant

English: As expectorant takes only 4 or 5 tablespoons each hour, to avoid vomiting.

Spanish: Como expectorante se toman únicamente 4 ó 5 cucharadas cada hora, para evitar que se produzcan vómitos.

564. Gotas para los ojos

Translation: eye drops

English: Often, you'll be given eyedrops to open up (dilate) your pupils.

Spanish: Con frecuencia, se le administran gotas para los ojos para abrir (dilatar) las pupilas.

565. Hormonas

Translation: hormones

English: We need to stabilize her human hormone levels and quick.

Spanish: Tenemos que estabilizar rapidamnete sus niveles de hormonas.

DAY 57

MEDICATIONS – MEDICAMENTOS

566. Ibuprofeno
Translation: ibuprophen
English: Use medicines such as ibuprofen or acetaminophen to ease pain.
Spanish: Se pueden utilizar analgésicos como ibuprofeno o paracetamol para aliviar el dolor.

567. Insulina
Translation: insulin
English: It must only be used in insulin pumps suitable for this insulin.
Spanish: Sólo debe utilizarse bombas de insulina adecuadas para esta insulina.

568. Yodo
Translation: iodine
English: You will also find several iodine tablets in your weekly rations.
Spanish: También encontrarán tabletas de yodo en sus raciones semanales.

569. Hierro
Translation: iron
English: Young lady, you're not getting enough iron.
Spanish: Jovencita, no consume suficiente hierro.

570. Laxante, purgante, "purga"
Translation: laxative, purgative
English: No, that was only a laxative, Helena.
Spanish: No, era solo un laxante, Helena.

571. Linimento
Translation: liniment
English: I've got some liniment.
Spanish: Tengo algo de linimento.

572. Pastillas para chupar
Translation: lozenges
English: Suck on hard candies or throat lozenges.
Spanish: Chupar dulces duros o pastillas para la garganta.

573. Atomizador nasal
Translation: nasal spray
English: Don't forget your nasal spray.
Spanish: No te olvides de tu atomizador nasal.

574. Ung ento, pomada, untamiento
Translation: ointment
English: They prescribed him an ointment to alleviate the burn.
Spanish: Le recetaron un ungüento para aliviar la quemadura.

575. Medicamento que no requiere receta m dica
Translation: over the counter medication
English: Tell your doctor about all the prescription and over-the-counter medications you use.
Spanish: Hable con su médico acerca de todas las recetas y de los medicamentos sin receta que ha consumido.

DAY 58

MEDICATIONS – MEDICAMENTOS

576. Oxitoc n
Translation:
English: oxytocin

577. Medicina para el dolor
Translation:
English: pain killer

578. Pareg rico, narc tico
Translation:
English: paregoric

579. Penicilina
Translation:
English: penicillin

580. Pastilla, p ldora
Translation:
English: pill

581. Placebo
Translation:
English: placebo

582. Vitaminas prenatales
Translation:
English: prenatal vitamins

583. Receta m dica, prescripci n
Translation:
English: **prescription**

584. Medicamento que requiere receta m dica
Translation:
English: **prescription drug**

585. Sedante, calmante
Translation:
English: **sedative**

DAY 59

MEDICATIONS – MEDICAMENTOS

586. Pastillas para dormir
Translation:
English: **sleeping pills**

587. Sales arom ticas
Translation:
English: **smelling salts**

588. Estimulante
Translation:
English: **stimulant**

589. Sulfa
Translation:
English: **sulfa**

590. Supositorio
Translation:
English: **suppository**

591. Jarabe
Translation:
English: **syrup**

592. Tableta
Translation:
English: **tablet**

593. T nico
Translation:
English: tonic

594. Tranquilizante, calmante
Translation:
English: tranquilizer

595. Vasodilatador
Translation:
English: vasodilator

596. Vitaminas
Translation:
English: vitamins

DAY 60

INSTRUCTIONS FOR TAKING MEDICATIONS - INSTRUCCIONES PARA TOMAR MEDICAMENTOS

597. Tome esta medicina
Translation:
English: Take this medicine:

- _____ times a day
- every _____ hours
- dissolved in water
- when you get up in the morning
- before you go to bed
- before each meal
- with each meal
- after each meal
- every other day
- with plenty of water

- _____ veces al día
- cada _____ horas
- disuelta en agua
- al levantarse por la mañana
- antes de acostarse
- antes de cada comida
- con cada comida
- después de cada comida
- cada tercer día, "un día sí y otro no"
- con mucha agua

598. No tome esta medicina con el est mago vacio
Translation:
English: Do not take this medication on an empy stomach

599. Este medicamento puede causar somnolencia/sue o
Translation:
English: This medication might cause drowsiness

600. Coloque una tableta debajo de su lengua cuando sienta el dolor
Translation:
English: Place one tablet under your tongue when you feel the pain

601. No beba alcohol mientras est tomando esta medicina
Translation:
English: Do not drink alcohol while taking this medication

602. No se exponga directamente al sol mientras est tomando este medicamento
Translation:
English: Do not expose yourself to direct sunlight while taking this medication

603. Aseg rese de terminar toda la medicina antes de dejar de tomarla
Translation:
English: Make sure you finish all the medicine before you stop taking it

604. Mant ngala refrigerada
Translation:
English: Keep it refrigerated

605. Ag tela bien antes de tomarla
Translation:
English: Shake well before taking it

606. Mant ngala fuera del alcance de los ni os
Translation:
English: Keep it out of reach of children

DAY 61

COMMUNICABLE DISEASES - ENFERMEDADES TRANSMISIBLES

607. Vacunas
Translation:
English: vaccines

608. Prevenibles por vacunaci n
Translation:
English: preventible diseases

609. Difteria
Translation:
English: diphtheria

610. Gripe
Translation:
English: flu

611. Hepatitis A, B, C
Translation:
English: hepatitis A, B, C

612. Enfermedad por Hib
Translation:
English: hib disease

613. Sarampi n
Translation:
English: measles

614. Paperas, parotiditis, "paper n", "chanza", "orejones"
Translation:
English: mumps

615. Pertusis, tos ferina, "tos ahogona", "tos ahogadora", "tos chichimeca", "tos de andancia", "coqueluche"
Translation:
English: pertussis, whooping cough

616. Enfermedad por pneumococo
Translation:
English: pneumococcal disease

617. Polio, par lisis infantil
Translation:
English: polio

618. Viruela
Translation:
English: smallpox

619. Rub ola, sarampi n alem n, "alfombrilla"
Translation:
English: rubella, german measles

620. Varicela, "viruela loca"
Translation:
English: varicella, chickenpox

DAY 62

COMMUNICABLE DISEASES - ENFERMEDADES TRANSMISIBLES

621. Reacci n acelerada:
Translation:
English: accelerated reaction:
- immune   - inmune
- negative   - negativa
- positive   - positiva

622. Tejido adiposo, grasa subcut nea, "la grasita debajo de la piel"
Translation:
English: adipose tissue

623. Bacteria
Translation:
English: bacteria

624. Refuerzo
Translation:
English: booster shot

625. Calibre, grosor de la aguja
Translation:
English: caliber (of the needle)

626. Contagio, contagioso, "que se pega"
Translation:
English: contagion, contagious

627. Deltoides
Translation:
English: deltoid

628. Jeringa desechable/descartable
Translation:
English: disposable syringe

629. Dosis
Translation:
English: dose

630. Respuesta inmunol gica
Translation:
English: immune response

631. Sistema inmunol gico, sistema de defensa
Translation:
English: immune system

632. Inmunizaci n, vacunaci n
Translation:
English: immunization

633. Comprobante de inmunizaci n, tarjeta de vacunas, carnet de vacunaci n
Translation:
English: immunization record

634. C lula inmunol gica
Translation:
English: immunologic cell

DAY 63

COMMUNICABLE DISEASES - ENFERMEDADES TRANSMISIBLES

635. Inyecci n
Translation:
English: injection:
- intramuscular   - intramuscular (en el músculo)
- intravenous   - intravenosa (en la vena)
- subcutaneous   - subcutánea (por debajo de la piel)

636. Inoculaci n
Translation:
English: inoculation

637. Aguja
Translation:
English: needle

638. Largo de la aguja
Translation:
English: needle length

639. Tama o de la aguja
Translation:
English: needle size

640. Vacuna oral
Translation:
English: oral vaccine

641. Brote, epidemia
Translation:
English: outbreak

642. Reacci n
Translation:
English: reaction

643. Riesgo
Translation:
English: risk

644. Prueba serol gica
Translation:
English: serological test

645. Vacuna, inyecci n, "piquete"
Translation:
English: shot

DAY 64

COMMUNICABLE DISEASES - ENFERMEDADES TRANSMISIBLES

646. Efecto secundario
Translation:
English: side effect

647. Jeringa
Translation:
English: syringe

648. Prendi /peg la vacuna
Translation:
English: the vaccine took

649. Vacunar
Translation:
English: to immunize

650. Prevenir
Translation:
English: to prevent

651. Vacunaci n
Translation:
English: vaccination

652. Brote, epidemia
Translation:
English: outbreak

653. Frasco, ampolleta
Translation:
English: vial

654. Riesgo
Translation:
English: risk

655. Infecci n viral
Translation:
English: viral infection

DAY 65

MATERNAL AND CHILD HEALTH - ATENCIÓN MÉDICA MATERNA E INFANTIL

656. Aborto (provocado)
Translation:
English: abortion

657. Desprendimiento prematuro de la placenta
Translation:
English: abruptio placentae

658. Escala de Agpar, prueba al momento de nacer
Translation:
English: Agpar test

659. Amniocentesis
Translation:
English: amniocentesis, "amnio"

660. L quido amni tico
Translation:
English: amniotic fluid

661. Anestesia
Translation:
English: anesthesia

662. Beb , nen (a), ni o(a)
Translation:
English: baby

663. Dolor de espalda durante el parto
Translation:
English: back labor

664. Dolores de espalda/de cintura
Translation:
English: back pains

665. Bolsa/fuente de aguas
Translation:
English: bag of waters

DAY 66

MATERNAL AND CHILD HEALTH - ATENCIÓN MÉDICA MATERNA E INFANTIL

666. Desecho con sangre
Translation:
English: bloody show

667. Presentaci n de nalgas/"trasero"
Translation:
English: breech presentation

668. Escala de Agpar, prueba al momento de nacer
Translation:
English: Agpar test

669. Ces rea
Translation:
English: cesarean section, "C section"

670. Gestaci n, embarazo
Translation:
English: childbearing

671. Parto, nacimiento, alumbramiento
Translation:
English: childbirth

672. Concepci n
Translation:
English: conception

673. Contracciones
Translation:
English: contractions

674. Antojos
Translation:
English: cravings

675. Sala de parto
Translation:
English: delivery room

DAY 67

MATERNAL AND CHILD HEALTH - ATENCIÓN MÉDICA MATERNA E INFANTIL

676. Dilataci n de la cervix
Translation:
English: cervical dilatation

677. Duchas/lavados vaginales
Translation:
English: douches

678. Fecha estimada de parto, "fecha en la que se alivia"
Translation:
English: due date

679. Eclampsia
Translation:
English: eclampsia

680. Embarazo ect pico
Translation:
English: ectopic pregnancy

681. Embri n
Translation:
English: embryo

682. Endometritis
Translation:
English: endometritis

683. Epidural
Translation:
English: epidural

684. Episiotom a
Translation:
English: episiotomy

685. Expulsi n
Translation:
English: expulsion

DAY 68

MATERNAL AND CHILD HEALTH - ATENCIÓN MÉDICA MATERNA E INFANTIL

686. Parto falso
Translation:
English: **false labor**

687. Sufrimiento fetal
Translation:
English: **fetal distress**

688. Monitoreo fetal
Translation:
English: **fetal monitoring**

689. Feto
Translation:
English: **fetus**

690. cido f lico
Translation:
English: **folic acid**

691. Forceps
Translation:
English: **forceps**

692. Embarazo a t rmino/completo
Translation:
English: **full-term pregnancy**

693. Ginec logo(a)
Translation:
English: **gynecologist**

694. Presentaci n de cabeza
Translation:
English: **head presentation**

695. Gemelos
Translation:
English: **identical twins**

DAY 69

MATERNAL AND CHILD HEALTH - ATENCIÓN MÉDICA MATERNA E INFANTIL

696. Inducci n
Translation:
English: induction

697. Intravenoso(a)
Translation:
English: intravenous, IV

698. Parto, trabajo de parto
Translation:
English: labor

699. Posiciones durante el parto
Translation:
English: labor positions

700. Loquios
Translation:
English: lochia

701. Partera, comadrona, "abuela", "facultativa", "sacadora"
Translation:
English: midwife

702. Aborto espont neo/natural/no deseado, "p rdida", "mal parto", "brote", "cama chica", "contrariedad", "descarrilamiento", "mala cama"

Translation:

English: **miscarriage**

703. Parto natural

Translation:

English: **natural childbirth**

704. Madre primeriza, nul para

Translation:

English: **new mother**

705. Placenta

Translation:

English: **placenta**

DAY 70

MATERNAL AND CHILD HEALTH - ATENCIÓN MÉDICA MATERNA E INFANTIL

706. Embarazo
Translation:
English: pregnancy

707. Prueba de embarazo
Translation:
English: pregnancy test

708. Antes del parto
Translation:
English: prelabor

709. Empujar, pujar
Translation:
English: push downwards

710. Etapas del parto
Translation:
English: stages of childbirth

711. Puntos, puntadas, "coser"
Translation:
English: stitches

712. Desgarre, desgarramiento
Translation:
English: tear

**713. Estar embarazada, esperando, pre ada, en cinta, "en estado",
"enferma de ni o", "de encago", "cargada", "pesada"**
Translation:
English: to be pregnant

714. Concebir
Translation:
English: to conceive

715. Dar a luz, tener el beb , parir, "aliviarse", "mejorarse", "componerse"
Translation:
English: to deliver, to give birth

DAY 71

MATERNAL AND CHILD HEALTH - ATENCIÓN MÉDICA MATERNA E INFANTIL

716. Cordón umbilical
Translation:
English: umbilical cord

717. Muestra de orina
Translation:
English: urine sample

718. Examen de orina
Translation:
English: urinalysis

719. Postparto
Translation:
English: postpartum

720. Dolores después del parto
Translation:
English: after pains

721. Defecto de nacimiento
Translation:
English: birth defect

722. Atiborramiento de senos
Translation:
English: breast engorgment

723. Leche materna
Translation:
English: breast milk

724. Bomba para senos
Translation:
English: breast pump

725. Amamantar, dar el pecho, lactar, dar de mamar, "dar chichi/chiche/chuchu"
Translation:
English: breast-feed, nurse

DAY 72

MATERNAL AND CHILD HEALTH - ATENCIÓN MÉDICA MATERNA E INFANTIL

726. Circuncisi n
Translation:
English: circumcision

727. lactancia
Translation:
English: lactation

728. Mastitis, infecci n de los senos
Translation:
English: mastitis, breast infection

729. Maternidad
Translation:
English: maternity

730. Gl ndulas mamarias
Translation:
English: milk glands

731. Reci n nacido
Translation:
English: newborn

732. Paternidad
Translation:
English: paternity

733. Depresi n postnatal
Translation:
English: postpartum depression, "baby blues"

734. Prematuro, antes de tiempo, "sietemesino", "sietilo"
Translation:
English: premature

735. Recuperaci n
Translation:
English: recovery

DAY 73

MATERNAL AND CHILD HEALTH - ATENCIÓN MÉDICA MATERNA E INFANTIL

736. Toallas sanitarias/higi nicas, cintur n sanitario, "Kotex"
Translation:
English: sanitary napkins

737. Pezones adoloridos
Translation:
English: sore nipples

738. Tampones
Translation:
English: tampons

739. Enganchar
Translation:
English: to latch on, hook

740. Chupar
Translation:
English: to suck

741. Peso al nacer
Translation:
English: weight at birth

742. Cuidado infantil
Translation:
English: infant care

743. Infancia, ni ez
Translation:
English: **childhood**

744. Puerperio, "cuarentena"
Translation:
English: **puerperium**

745. F rmula, leche en polvo
Translation:
English: **formula**

DAY 74

SEXUALLY TRANSMITTED DISEASES
ENFERMEDADES de TRANSMISIÓN SEXUAL (ETS)

746. S filis, "sangre mala"
Translation:
English: syphilis, "bad blood"

747. Chancro
Translation:
English: chancroid

748. Clamidia
Translation:
English: chlamydia

749. Condilomas
Translation:
English: condyloma, genital warts

750. Enfermedad p lvica inflamatoria
Translation:
English: Pelvic Inflammatory Disease (PID)

751. Entameba
Translation:
English: entamoeba

752. Gonorrea
Translation:
English: gonorrhea

753. H rpes genital
Translation:
English: **genital herpes**

754. Ladilla
Translation:
English: **crabs**

755. Piojo del pubis
Translation:
English: **pubic lice**

DAY 75

756. Abstinencia , no tener relaciones sexuales
Translation:
English: abstinence, not having sex

757. Aplicador
Translation:
English: applicator

758. Control de natalidad
Translation:
English: birth control

759. Implante anticonceptivo
Translation:
English: birth control implant

760. M todo anticonceptivo/contraceptivo/de control de natalidad
Translation:
English: birth control method

761. Inyecci n anticonceptiva
Translation:
English: birth control shot

762. Capa/capuch n cervical
Translation:
English: cervical cap

763. Edad reproductiva
Translation:
English: childbearing age

764. Cond n, preservativo, profil ctico, "gorrito", "capucha", "globito"
Translation:
English: **condom, rubber, preservative**

765. Diafragma
Translation:
English: **diaphragm**

DAY 76

FAMILY PLANNING - PLANIFICACION FAMILIAR

766. P ldora anticonceptiva de emergencia
Translation:
English: emergency contraception pill

767. Erecci n
Translation:
English: erection

768. Cond n femenino/de la mujer
Translation:
English: female condom

769. M todo de conocimiento de la fertilidad
Translation:
English: fertility awareness method

770. Moco, mucosidad
Translation:
English: mucus

771. Orgasmo, cl max
Translation:
English: orgasm

772. Ovulaci n, per odo f rtil
Translation:
English: ovulation, fertile period

773. Esperma
Translation:
English: sperm

774. Espermicida
Translation:
English: spermicide

775. Vasectom a, esterilizaci n del hombre
Translation:
English: vasectomy

DAY 77

DENTAL HEALTH - SALUD DENTAL

776. Premolares, bic spides
Translation:
English: **bicuspids**

777. Caninos, colmillos
Translation:
English: **canine, eyetooth**

778. Incisivos, dientes delanteros
Translation:
English: **incisors, front teeth**

779. Molares, muelas
Translation:
English: **molars**

780. Tercer molar, "muela del juicio", "muela cordal"
Translation:
English: **wisdom tooth**

781. Alv olo
Translation:
English: **alveolus, tooth socket**

782. Capilares
Translation:
English: **capillaries**

783. Corona
Translation:
English: **crown**

784. Esmalte
Translation:
English: enamel

785. Ra z
Translation:
English: root, fang

DAY 78

DENTAL HEALTH - SALUD DENTAL

786. Absceso, postemilla
Translation:
English: abscess

787. Caries del biber n
Translation:
English: baby bottle tooth decay

788. Cavidad, "picada"
Translation:
English: cavity

789. Caries, "dientes picados"
Translation:
English: tooth decay

790. Gingivitis
Translation:
English: gingivitis

791. Enfermedad periodontal
Translation:
English: periodontal disease

792. Mal aliento
Translation:
English: bad breath

793. Morder, mordida
Translation:
English: bite

794. Blanqueamiento
Translation:
English: bleaching, whitening

795. Cerdas
Translation:
English: bristles

DAY 79

DENTAL HEALTH - SALUD DENTAL

796. Dientes salidos
Translation:
English: buck teeth

797. Masticar, mascar
Translation:
English: to chew

798. Odontolog a/dentister a cosm tica
Translation:
English: cosmetic dentistry

799. Dientes da ados
Translation:
English: damaged teeth

800. Frenillos, frenos dentales
Translation:
English: dental braces

801. Cemento dental
Translation:
English: dental cement

802. Limpieza dental
Translation:
English: dental cleaning

803. Hilo/seda/cord n dental
Translation:
English: dental floss

804. Espejo dental
Translation:
English: dental mirror

805. Silla de dentista
Translation:
English: dentist's chair

DAY 80

DENTAL HEALTH - SALUD DENTAL

806. Dentadura postiza, pr tesis dental, caja de dientes, placa
Translation:
English: **denture, false teeth**

807. Torno dental, fresa
Translation:
English: **drill**

808. Empaste, relleno, "tapadura", "calza"
Translation:
English: **filling**

809. Fluorizaci n
Translation:
English: **fluoridation**

810. Fluoruro, fl or
Translation:
English: **fluoride**

811. Tenazas
Translation:
English: **forceps**

812. Hacer g rgaras
Translation:
English: **gargle**

813. Oro
Translation:
English: **gold**

814. Enjuague bucal
Translation:
English: mouth rinse/wash

815. Protector de boca
Translation:
English: mouth guard

DAY 81

DENTAL HEALTH - SALUD DENTAL

816. Paladar
Translation:
English: palate

817. Dientes permanentes
Translation:
English: permanent teeth

818. Placa bacteriana
Translation:
English: plaque

819. Porcelana
Translation:
English: porcelain

820. Pr tesis
Translation:
English: prosthesis

821. Resina
Translation:
English: resin

822. Enjuagar, enjuague
Translation:
English: to rinse

823. Plata
Translation:
English: silver

824. Saliva
Translation:
English: **saliva**

825. Sellante
Translation:
English: **sealant**

DAY 82

DENTAL HEALTH - SALUD DENTAL

826. Dientes sensibles
Translation:
English: sensitive teeth

827. Dentadura
Translation:
English: set of teeth

828. Escupidera
Translation:
English: spittoon

829. Sarro
Translation:
English: tartar

830. Cepillo de dientes
Translation:
English: toothbrush

831. Pasta/crema de dientes, dent frico
Translation:
English: toothpaste

832. Palillo de dientes, mondadientes, picadientes
Translation:
English: toothpick

833. Anestesia total/general
Translation:
English: total anesthesia

834. Pinzas
Translation:
English: tweezers

835. Sin dientes, mueco, "chimuelo", "cholco"
Translation:
English: without or missing teeth

DAY 83

ENVIRONMENTAL HEALTH - SALUD AMBIENTAL

836. Absorci n
Translation:
English: absorption

837. Agencia para Sustancias T xicas y Registro de Enfermedades
Translation:
English: Agency for Toxic Substances and Disease Registry (ATSDR)

838. Agentes
Translation:
English: agents

839. Contaminaci n del aire
Translation:
English: air pollution

840. Calidad del aire
Translation:
English: air quality

841. Ambiente, entorno
Translation:
English: ambient, environment, surroundings

842. Aire ambiental
Translation:
English: ambient air

843. Monitoreo biol gico
Translation:
English: biological monitoring

844. Bioterrorismo
Translation:
English: bioterrorism

845. Nivel de plomo en la sangre
Translation:
English: blood lead level

DAY 84

ENVIRONMENTAL HEALTH - SALUD AMBIENTAL

846. Cadmio
Translation:
English: cadmium

847. Mon xido de carbono
Translation:
English: carbon monoxide

848. Cancer geno(a), carcin geno(a)
Translation:
English: carcinogen

849. Estudio de caso
Translation:
English: case study

850. Centros de Control y Prevenci n de Enfermedades
Translation:
English: Centers for Disease Control and Prevention (CDC)

851. Qu micos
Translation:
English: chemicals

852. Cr nico(a)
Translation:
English: chronic

853. Investigaci n de sectores
Translation:
English: cluster investigation

854. Salud de la comunidad
Translation:
English: community health

855. Concentraci n
Translation:
English: concentration

DAY 85

ENVIRONMENTAL HEALTH - SALUD AMBIENTAL

856. Contaminante
Translation:
English: contaminant

857. Aire contaminado
Translation:
English: contaminated air

858. Agua contaminada
Translation:
English: contaminated water

859. Planeaci n de contingencia
Translation:
English: contingency planning

860. Escama de la piel
Translation:
English: skin flake, psoriasis

861. D rmico
Translation:
English: dermal

862. Diox n
Translation:
English: dioxin

863. Registro de enfermedades
Translation:
English: disease registry

864. Drenaje
Translation:
English: **drainage**

865. Polvo
Translation:
English: **dust**

DAY 86

ENVIRONMENTAL HEALTH - SALUD AMBIENTAL

866. Respuesta de emergencia
Translation:
English: emergency response

867. Medio ambiente, entorno
Translation:
English: environment

868. Ambiental, del medio ambiente
Translation:
English: environmental

869. Agencia de Protecci n del Medio Ambiente
Translation:
English: Environmental Protection Agency (EPA)

870. Epidemiolog a
Translation:
English: epidemiology

871. Evaluaci n de exposici n
Translation:
English: exposure assessment

872. Ruta de exposici n
Translation:
English: exposure route

873. Bacteria coliforme fecal
Translation:
English: fecal coliform bacteria

874. Primeros en responder
Translation:
English: first responders

875. Enfermedades causadas por alimentos
Translation:
English: food-borne illnesses

DAY 87

ENVIRONMENTAL HEALTH - SALUD AMBIENTAL

876. Pelo de animal
Translation:
English: fur

877. Agua subterr nea
Translation:
English: groundwater

878. Peligro
Translation:
English: danger, hazard

879. Sustancia peligrosa
Translation:
English: hazardous substance

880. Evaluaci n de salud
Translation:
English: health assessment

881. Educaci n de salud
Translation:
English: health education

882. Investigaci n de salud
Translation:
English: health investigation

883. Metales pesados
Translation:
English: heavy metals

884. Desechos peligrosos del hogar
Translation:
English: household hazardous waste

885. Humedad
Translation:
English: humidity

DAY 88

ENVIRONMENTAL HEALTH - SALUD AMBIENTAL

886. Higiene
Translation:
English: hygiene

887. Incidencia
Translation:
English: incidence

888. Indicadores
Translation:
English: indicators

889. Dentro, adentro, interior
Translation:
English: indoors

890. Enfermedad infecciosa
Translation:
English: infectious disease

891. Observaci n m dica, monitoreo m dico
Translation:
English: medical monitoring

892. Mercurio
Translation:
English: mercury

893. Metabolismo
Translation:
English: metabolism

894. Contaminaci n microbiol gica
Translation:
English: microbiological contamination

895. Nivel m nimo de riesgo
Translation:
English: minimal risk level (MRL)

DAY 89

ENVIRONMENTAL HEALTH - SALUD AMBIENTAL

896.   caro
Translation:
English: mite

897. Moho
Translation:
English: mold

898. Monitoreo
Translation:
English: monitoring

899. Morbosidad
Translation:
English: morbidity

900. Mortalidad
Translation:
English: mortality

901. Exterior, afuera, al aire libre
Translation:
English: outdoors

902. Ozono
Translation:
English: ozone

903. Part culas
Translation:
English: particles

904. Pesticida
Translation:
English: pesticide

905. Residuos de pesticida
Translation:
English: pesticide residues

DAY 90

ENVIRONMENTAL HEALTH - SALUD AMBIENTAL

906. Mascota
Translation:
English: pet

907. Polen
Translation:
English: pollen

908. Poblaci n en riesgo
Translation:
English: population at risk

909. Prevalencia
Translation:
English: prevalence

910. Salud p blica
Translation:
English: public health

911. Remediar, corrregir, arreglar
Translation:
English: remediation

912. Enfermedades repiratorias
Translation:
English: respiratory diseases

913. Reusar
Translation:
English: to reuse

914. Agua segura
Translation:
English: **safe water**

915. Sanidad
Translation:
English: **sanitation**

DAY 91

ENVIRONMENTAL HEALTH - SALUD AMBIENTAL

916. Aguas residuales/negras/servidas
Translation:
English: sewage

917. Alcantarilla, cloaca
Translation:
English: sewer

918. Humo
Translation:
English: smoke

919. Desecho s lido
Translation:
English: solid waste

920. Espora
Translation:
English: spore

921. Di xido de sulfuro
Translation:
English: sulfur dioxide

922. Agua de la superficie
Translation:
English: surface water

923. Vigilancia
Translation:
English: surveillance

924. T xico
Translation:
English: **toxic**

925. Toxicolog a
Translation:
English: **toxicology**

DAY 92

ENVIRONMENTAL HEALTH - SALUD AMBIENTAL

926. Provocadores, causantes
Translation:
English: triggers

927. Vol til
Translation:
English: volatile

928. Compuestos org nicos vol tiles
Translation:
English: volatile organic compounds (VOCs)

929. Agua residual
Translation:
English: wastewater

930. Tratamiento de aguas residuales
Translation:
English: wastewater treatment

931. Contaminaci n del agua
Translation:
English: water pollution

932. Calidad del agua
Translation:
English: water quality

933. Lugar, sitio
Translation:
English: site, place

934. Smog
Translation:
English: smog

935. Lugar de investigaci n
Translation:
English: investigation site

DAY 93

ENFERMEDADES CRONICAS - CHRONIC DISEASES

936. presi n arterial, tensi n
Translation:
English: **blood preassure**

937. az car en la sangre, glucosa
Translation:
English: **blood sugar, glucose**

938. m quina para medir el az car/glucosa en la sangre
Translation:
English: **blood sugar/glucose meter**

939. colesterol
Translation:
English: **cholesterol**

940. diabetes, "betis", az car en la sangre", "orina dulce"
Translation:
English: **diabetes**

941. educaci n sobre la diabetes
Translation:
English: **diabetes education**

942. pastillas para la diabetes
Translation:
English: **diabetes pills**

943. automanejo de la diabetes, cuidar de su diabetes
Translation:
English: **diabetes self-management**

944. ex men de los ojos con dilataci n
Translation:
English: **dilated eye exam**

945. ex men de los pies
Translation:
English: **foot exam**

DAY 94

ENFERMEDADES CRONICAS - CHRONIC DISEASES

946. hemoglobina A1C
Translation:
English: hemoglobin A1C

947. hiperglicemia (az car alta en la sangre)
Translation:
English: hyperglycemia (high sugar level)

948. hipoglicemia (az car baja en la sangre)
Translation:
English: blood sugar/glucose meter

949. insulina
Translation:
English: insulin

950. insulinodependiente, dependiente de la insulina
Translation:
English: insulin-dependent

951. prueba de los ri ones
Translation:
English: kidney test

952. diab tico(a), persona con diabetes
Translation:
English: person with diabetes

953. actividad f sica
Translation:
English: physical activity

954. pre-diabetes
Translation:
English: **pre-diabetes**

955. hacer ejercicio regularmente
Translation:
English: **regular exercise**

DAY 95

ENFERMEDADES CRONICAS - CHRONIC DISEASES

956. aire
Translation:
English: air

957. filtro de aire
Translation:
English: air filter

958. v as respiratorias/a reas
Translation:
English: airways

959. al rgeno, alerg nico
Translation:
English: allergen

960. al rgico(a)
Translation:
English: allergic

961. alergia
Translation:
English: allergy

962. anticolin rgico
Translation:
English: anti-colinergic

963. anti-inflamatorio
Translation:
English: anti-inflammatory

964. asma, "ansia", "ansiedad", "acecido", "ahogamiento", "ahogui", "apretamiento de la pechera", "cansancio de aliento", "hoguido"
Translation:
English: asthma

965. ataque de asma
Translation:
English: asthma attack

DAY 96

ENFERMEDADES CRONICAS - CHRONIC DISEASES

966. tos asm tica
Translation:
English: asthma cough

967. episodio asm tico
Translation:
English: asthma episode

968. plan de asma
Translation:
English: asthma plan

969. bronquitis asm tica
Translation:
English: asthmatic bronchitis

970. soplar, exhalar
Translation:
English: blow out

971. inhalar, respirar hacia dentro, inspirar
Translation:
English: to breath in

972. respirar
Translation:
English: to breath

973. problema respiratorio
Translation:
English: breathing problem

974. asma bronquial
Translation:
English: bronchial asthma

975. pomo, bote
Translation:
English: canister

DAY 97

ENFERMEDADES CRONICAS - CHRONIC DISEASES

976. cr nico(a)
Translation:
English: chronic

977. enfermedad cr nica obstructiva pulmonar
Translation:
English: chronic obstructive pulmonary disease (COPD)

978. compresor
Translation:
English: compressor

979. contraer
Translation:
English: contract

980. coticoesteroides
Translation:
English: corticoesteroids

981. dilatar
Translation:
English: dilate

982. efisema
Translation:
English: emphysema

983. humo de tabaco ambiental
Translation:
English: environmental tobacco smoke (ETS)

984. exacerbaci n, agravamiento
Translation:
English: exacerbation

985. sistema inmunol gico/de defensa
Translation:
English: immune system

DAY 98

ENFERMEDADES CRONICAS - CHRONIC DISEASES

986. inhalar, respirar hacia dentro, inspirar
Translation:
English: to inhale

987. medicina inhalada
Translation:
English: inhaled medicine

988. nebulizador, m quina de vapor
Translation:
English: nebulizer

989. flujo m ximo pulmonar, funci n pulmonar
Translation:
English: peak flow

990. enfermedad reactiva de las v as respiratorias
Translation:
English: reactive airway disease (RAD)

991. retracci n de la piel del pecho
Translation:
English: sucking in the chest skin

992. corto(a)/falta de aire, ahogo
Translation:
English: shortness of breath

993. zonas de flujo m ximo pulmonar
Translation:
English: peak flow zones:
- green/ under control zone
- yellow/ caution zone
- red/ danger zone
- verde/ zona bajo control
- amarilla/ zona de precaución
- roja/ zona de peligro

994. terapia alternativa
Translation:
English: alternative therapy

995. biopsia
Translation:
English: biopsy

DAY 99

ENFERMEDADES CRONICAS - CHRONIC DISEASES

996. auto ex men de los senos
Translation:
English: breast self-exam

997. estern n
Translation:
English: breastbone

998. c ncer
Translation:
English: cancer:
- breast   - de seno
- cervical   - cervical
- ovarian   - de los ovarios
- prostatic   - de la próstata

999. cancer geno(a), carcin geno(a)
Translation:
English: carcinogen

1000. quimioterapia
Translation:
English: chemotherapy

1001. colposcop a
Translation:
English: colposcopy

1002. displasia
Translation:
English: dysplasia

1003. fibroma
Translation:
English: **fibroma**

1004. histerectom a
Translation:
English: **hysterectomy**

1005. c ncer invasivo
Translation:
English: **invasive cancer**

DAY 100

ENFERMEDADES CRONICAS - CHRONIC DISEASES

1006. terapia hormonal
Translation:
English: hormone therapy

1007. leucemia, c ncer de la sangre
Translation:
English: leukemia, blood cancer

1008. mamograma, mamograf a
Translation:
English: mammogram, mammography

1009. met stasis
Translation:
English: metastasis

1010. prueba/ex men PAP (Papanicolaou), prueba del c ncer
Translation:
English: PAP exam

1011. pr tesis
Translation:
English: prosthesis

1012. radioterapia
Translation:
English: radiotherapy

1013. recurrente, que vuelve a aparecer
Translation:
English: recurrence

1014. tumor
Translation:
English: tumor:
- benign   - benigno
- malignant   - maligno

1015. tumorectom a
Translation:
English: lumpectomy

DIALOGUES

DOLOR ABDOMINAL – ABDOMINAL PAIN

Doctor: Tengo entendido que le duele el estómago.

Patient: Sí.

Doctor: ¿El dolor es constante, o viene y se va?

Patient: Viene y se va.

Doctor: ¿Está libre de dolor a veces?

Patient: Sí.

Doctor: ¿El dolor le viaja a otra parte del cuerpo?

Patient: No.

Doctor: ¿Se pone peor cuando come?

Patient: Sí.

Doctor: ¿Eructa o expulsa gases?

Patient: Sí, las dos cosas.

Doctor: Le voy a examinar el vientre.

ABDOMINAL PAIN

Doctor: I understand that your stomach has been hurting.

Patient: Yes

Doctor: Is the pain constant or does it come and go?

Patient: It comes and goes.

Doctor: Are there times when you are free of pain?

Patient: Yes.

Doctor: Does the pain travel to another part of your body?

Patient: No.

Doctor: Does eating make it worse?

Patient: Yes.

Doctor: Are you burping or passing gas?

Patient: Yes, both.

Doctor: I'm going to examine your abdomen.

DOLOR DE LA ESPALDA – BACK PAIN

Doctor: ¿Recuerda alguna lesión que le haya causado el dolor?

Patient: No.

Doctor: ¿Hace movimientos repetitivos en el trabajo o en la casa?

Patient: No, no en realidad.

Doctor: ¿El dolor le baja a la nalga o por la pierna?

Patient: Sí, por la pierna.

Doctor: ¿Siente entumecimiento, debilidad o hormigueo en las piernas?

Patient: No, sólo me duele.

Doctor: ¿Hay algún movimiento que empeore el dolor?

Patient: Me duele cuando me siento.

Doctor: ¿Toma alguna medicina para el dolor?

Patient: No.

Doctor: Por favor, póngase de pie para verla caminar.

BACK PAIN

Doctor: Do you remember an injury that caused the pain?

Patient: No.

Doctor: Do you perform repetitive movements at work or at home?

Patient: No, not really.

Doctor: Does the pain travel to your buttock or down your leg?

Patient: Yes, down my leg.

Doctor: Do you have any tingling, numbness, or weakness in your legs?

Patient: No, it just hurts.

Doctor: Is there a certain movement that makes it worse?

Patient: It hurts when I sit.

Doctor: Are you taking any medications for the pain?

Patient: No.

Doctor: Please stand up so that I can watch you walk.

DOLOR DE PECHO – CHEST PAIN

Doctor: Por favor, muéstreme dónde le duele exactamente.

Patient: Aquí.

Doctor: ¿Qué clase de dolor siente?

Patient: Es como presión en el pecho.

Doctor: ¿Qué estaba haciendo cuando le empezó el dolor?

Patient: Mirando la televisión.

Doctor: ¿Cuánto rato hace que tiene dolor?

Patient: Unas tres horas.

Doctor: ¿Le cuesta trabajo respirar?

Patient: Sí.

Doctor: ¿Tiene historial de enfermedad del corazón o presión alta?

Patient: Tengo la presión alta.

Doctor: Le voy a hacer un electrocardiograma.

CHEST PAIN

Doctor: Please point to the exact spot where it hurts.

Patient: Here.

Doctor: What does the pain feel like?

Patient: It's like pressure on my chest.

Doctor: What were you doing when the pain started?

Patient: Watching TV.

Doctor: How long have you had the pain?

Patient: For about three hours.

Doctor: Is it difficult to breathe?

Patient: Yes.

Doctor: Do you have a history of heart disease or high blood pressure?

Patient: I have high blood pressure.

Doctor: I'm going to do an electrocardiogram.

ESTREÑIMIENTO – CONSTIPATION

Doctor: ¿Tiene que esforzarse para mover los intestinos?

Patient: Sí.

Doctor: ¿Tiene el excremento duro?

Patient: Sí.

Doctor: ¿Tiene hemorroides?

Patient: No lo creo.

Doctor: ¿Ha notado sangre color rojo vivo?

Patient: Sí, un poco.

Doctor: ¿Tiene heces rojizas?

Patient: No.

Doctor: ¿Ha tomado laxantes o algún otro tratamiento sin receta?

Patient: Sí.

Doctor: ¿Le ayudó?

Patient: No, en realidad no.

Doctor: Vamos a necesitar una muestra de heces.

CONSTIPATION

Doctor: Do you have to strain to have a bowel movement?

Patient: Yes.

Doctor: Is your stool hard?

Patient: Yes.

Doctor: Do you have hemorrhoids?

Patient: I don't think so.

Doctor: Have you seen any bright red blood?

Patient: Yes, a little bit.

Doctor: Is your stool maroon in color?

Patient: No.

Doctor: Have you tried any over-the-counter treatments such as laxatives?

Patient: Yes.

Doctor: Was that helpful?

Patient: Not really.

Doctor: We're going to need a stool sample.

DEPRESIÓN – DEPRESSION

Doctor: Tengo entendido que se ha estado sintiendo triste.

Patient: Sí.

Doctor: ¿Cuánto tiempo hace que se siente así?

Patient: No sé. meses.

Doctor: ¿Sus sentimientos han afectado sus relaciones con familiares o compañeros de trabajo?

Patient: Con mi familia. No estoy trabajando.

Doctor: ¿Encuentra que se retira de las actividades con otras personas?

Patient: Sí.

Doctor: ¿Le cuesta trabajo quedarse dormido?

Patient: Sí.

Doctor: ¿Ha pensado en suicidarse?

Patient: No. Sí.

Doctor: ¿Ha pensado en cómo lo haría?

Patient: No, nunca lo he pensado.

Doctor: Gracias por compartir sus sentimientos conmigo. Vamos a hablar de algunas opciones de tratamiento.

DEPRESSION

Doctor: I understand that you have been feeling sad.

Patient: Yes.

Doctor: How long have you been feeling this way?

Patient: I don't know ... months.

Doctor: Have your feelings affected your relationship with your family or co-workers?

Patient: With my family ... I'm not working.

Doctor: Do you find yourself withdrawing from activities with other people?

Patient: Yes.

Doctor: Do you have trouble falling asleep?

Patient: Yes.

Doctor: Have you ever thought about killing yourself?

Patient: No ... yes.

Doctor: Have you thought about how you would do it?

Patient: No, I never thought about that.

Doctor: Thank you for sharing your feelings with me. Let's discuss some treatment options.

DIARREA – DIARRHEA

Doctor: ¿Cuánto tiempo hace que tiene diarrea?

Patient: Como una semana.

Doctor: ¿Cuántas veces al día tiene heces sueltas?

Patient: Dos o tres veces al día. Quizás cuatro veces.

Doctor: ¿Tiene cólicos?

Patient: Sí, un poco.

Doctor: ¿Se siente mejor después de ir al baño?

Patient: A veces. Sí, creo que sí.

Doctor: ¿Ha viajado recientemente?

Patient: Sí.

Doctor: ¿A dónde fue?

Patient: A Brooklyn.

Doctor: Por favor, acuéstese sobre la mesa pera examinarle el vientre.

DIARRHEA

Doctor: How long have you had diarrhea?

Patient: About a week.

Doctor: How many times a day do you have loose stools?

Patient: Two or three times every day. Maybe four times.

Doctor: Do you have any cramping?

Patient: Yes, a little bit.

Doctor: Is it better after using the bathroom?

Patient: Sometimes. Yes, I think so.

Doctor: Have you traveled recently?

Patient: Yes.

Doctor: Where did you go?

Patient: Cleveland.

Doctor: Please lie down on the exam table so I can examine your abdomen.

MAREO – DIZZINESS

Doctor: Veo en su hoja clínica que ha estado mareado.

Patient: Es verdad.

Doctor: ¿Se siente mareado?

Patient: Sí.

Doctor: ¿Cómo si se fuera a desmayar?

Patient: Sí.

Doctor: ¿Siente que la habitación gira a su alrededor?

Patient: A veces sí.

Doctor: Si se levanta de estar acostado, se marea?

Patient: Sí, es lo peor.

Doctor: ¿Hay alguna posición que no lo haga sentirse mareado?

Patient: Me siento mejor cuando estoy acostado.

Doctor: ¿Siente náuseas?

Patient: Sí, a veces.

Doctor: Lo voy a guiar hasta la mesa.

DIZZINESS

Doctor: I see from your chart that you have been feeling dizzy.

Patient: That's right.

Doctor: Do you feel light-headed?

Patient: Yes.

Doctor: Like you are going to pass out?

Patient: Yes.

Doctor: Do you feel like the room is spinning around you?

Patient: Sometimes, yes.

Doctor: If you get up from lying, does that make you dizzy?

Patient: Yes, that's when it's the worst.

Doctor: Is there a position where you are not dizzy?

Patient: It's better when I'm lying down.

Doctor: Do you feel nauseated?

Patient: Yes, sometimes.

Doctor: Let me help you to the exam table.

DOLOR de OIDOS – EARACHE

Doctor: ¿Le duelen los oídos?

Patient: Sólo el izquierdo.

Doctor: ¿Ha notado alguna supuración?

Patient: Sí.

Doctor: ¿Tiene dificultad al oír?

Patient: Un poco.

Doctor: ¿Ha ido a nadar recientemente?

Patient: El miércoles.

Doctor: Le voy a examinar los oídos.

Patient: Está bien.

Doctor: Por favor, gire la cabeza.

EARACHE

Doctor: Do your ears hurt?

Patient: Just the left one.

Doctor: Have you noticed any drainage?

Patient: Yes.

Doctor: Are you having difficulty hearing?

Patient: A little bit.

Doctor: Have you been swimming recently?

Patient: On Wednesday.

Doctor: I'm going to look in your ears.

Patient: Okay.

Doctor: Please turn your head ...

DOLOR DE CABEZA – HEADACHE

Doctor: Por favor indique dónde le duele la cabeza.

Patient: Aquí, en este lado.

Doctor: ¿El dolor le pulsa, o es más constante?

Patient: Constante.

Doctor: ¿Se despierta con dolor de cabeza?

Patient: Sí.

Doctor: ¿Mejora o empeora al progresar el día?

Patient: Quizás mejora un poco, pero empeora por la noche.

Doctor: ¿Cuánto tiempo hace que tiene este dolor de cabeza?

Patient: Como una semana.

Doctor: ¿Empeora progresivamente?

Patient: No lo creo.

Doctor: ¿Ha notado algún cambio en la vista?

Patient: No.

Doctor: Le voy a examinar la cabeza, los ojos, los oídos y el cuello.

HEADACHE

Doctor: Please point to where your head hurts.

Patient: Here, on the side.

Doctor: Is the pain throbbing or is it steadier?

Patient: Steady.

Doctor: Do you wake up with the headache?

Patient: Yes.

Doctor: Does it get better or worse as the day goes on?

Patient: Probably a little better, but worse at night.

Doctor: How long have you had this headache?

Patient: About a week.

Doctor: Is it getting progressively worse?

Patient: I don't think so.

Doctor: Have you noticed any change in your vision?

Patient: No.

Doctor: I'm going to examine you head, eyes, ears, and neck.

INSOMNIO – INSOMNIA

Doctor: ¿Le cuesta trabajo dormirse?

Patient: Sí.

Doctor: ¿Se siente descansado por la mañana?

Patient: No, me siento muy cansado.

Doctor: ¿Se queda dormido a veces durante el día?

Patient: Sí, a veces a la hora del almuerzo.

Doctor: ¿Está usted bajo mucho estrés?

Patient: Sí, en el trabajo.

Doctor: ¿Con qué frecuencia hace ejercicios?

Patient: No tengo mucho tiempo.

Doctor: Lo voy a examinar ahora. Por favor, siéntese sobre la mesa.

INSOMNIA

Doctor: Do you have trouble falling asleep?

Patient: Yes.

Doctor: Do you feel well rested in the morning?

Patient: No, I'm very tired.

Doctor: Do you sometimes doze off during the day?

Patient: Yes, sometimes at lunch.

Doctor: Are you under a lot of stress?

Patient: Yes, at work.

Doctor: How often do you exercise?

Patient: I don't have a lot of time.

Doctor: I'm going to examine you now. Please sit on the exam table.

DOLOR DE RODILLAS – KNEE PAIN

Doctor: ¿Cuánto tiempo hace que le duele la rodilla?

Patient: Hace unas dos semanas.

Doctor: ¿Se ha lastimado la rodilla alguna vez?

Patient: No, no lo creo.

Doctor: ¿Su trabajo requiere arrodillarse mucho?

Patient: Sí, mucho.

Doctor: ¿Le cede o se le dobla la rodilla al caminar?

Patient: No.

Doctor: ¿Se le traba a veces la rodilla de manera que no puede enderezar completamente la pierna?

Patient: No, sólo me duele.

Doctor: ¿Tiene la rodilla rígida cuando se levanta por la mañana?

Patient: Sí, es peor por la mañana.

Doctor: Le voy a examinar la rodilla parado, sentado y acostado.

KNEE PAIN

Doctor: How long has your knee been hurting you?

Patient: It's been a couple of weeks.

Doctor: Have you ever injured your knee?

Patient: No, I don't think so.

Doctor: Does your work require you to do a lot of kneeling?

Patient: Yes, a lot.

Doctor: Does your knee ever give way or buckle when you walk?

Patient: No.

Doctor: Does your knee sometimes lock so that you cannot completely straighten your leg?

Patient: No, it just hurts.

Doctor: Does your knee feel stiff when you get up in the morning?

Patient: Yes, it's worse in the morning.

Doctor: I'm going to examine your knee while you are standing, sitting, and lying down.

DOLOR de CUELLO – NECK PAIN

Doctor: ¿Hace cuánto tiempo que le duele?

Patient: Como una semana.

Doctor: ¿Le baja el dolor por los brazos?

Patient: No.

Doctor: ¿Qué movimiento lo empeora?

Patient: Cuando hago esto.

Doctor: ¿El dolor le impide dormir?

Patient: Sí.

Doctor: ¿Ha tenido problemas en el cuello antes?

Patient: Sí.

Doctor: ¿Le han hecho cirugía del cuello alguna vez?

Patient: No.

Doctor: Le voy a examinar el cuello y probarle los reflejos.

NECK PAIN

Doctor: How long have you had the pain?

Patient: About a week.

Doctor: Does the pain go down your arms?

Patient: No.

Doctor: What movement makes it worse?

Patient: When I do this.

Doctor: Does the pain prevent you from sleeping?

Patient: Yes.

Doctor: Have you had problems with your neck before?

Patient: Yes.

Doctor: Have you ever had neck surgery?

Patient: No.

Doctor: I am going to examine your neck and test your reflexes.

DOLOR DE OJOS / OJOS ROJOS – RED / PAINFUL EYE

Doctor: ¿Cuántos días hace que tiene rojo el ojo?

Patient: Cuatro días, doctor.

Doctor: ¿Cree que tiene algo en el ojo?

Patient: No lo creo.

Doctor: ¿Le molesta la luz en los ojos?

Patient: Quizás un poco.

Doctor: ¿Cuándo se hizo el último examen de los ojos?

Patient: No recuerdo.

Doctor: ¿Tiene glaucoma?

Patient: No.

Doctor: Le voy a examinar los ojos.

RED / PAINFUL EYE

Doctor: How many days has your eye been red?

Patient: Four days, doctor.

Doctor: Do you think you have something in your eye?

Patient: I don't think so.

Doctor: Does the light bother your eyes?

Patient: Maybe a little.

Doctor: When was your last eye exam?

Patient: I can't remember.

Doctor: Do you have glaucoma?

Patient: No.

Doctor: I'm going to examine your eyes.

FALTA DE ALIENTO – SHORTNESS OF BREATH

Doctor: ¿Cuánto tiempo hace que tiene dificultad al respirar?

Patient: Quizás dos semanas.

Doctor: ¿Le pasa todo el tiempo, o sólo cuando está haciendo algo?

Patient: Más cuando estoy haciendo algo.

Doctor: ¿Se despierta por la noche sin poder respirar?

Patient: No, no lo creo.

Doctor: ¿Resuella o tose?

Patient: Sí, un poco.

Doctor: ¿Tose con mucosidad?

Patient: Quizás un poco.

Doctor: ¿Tiene fiebre o escalofríos?

Patient: A veces escalofríos.

Doctor: Por favor, siéntese sobre la mesa para auscultarle los pulmones.

SHORTNESS OF BREATH

Doctor: How long have you been having difficulty breathing?

Patient: Maybe two weeks.

Doctor: Is it all the time, or only when you're doing something?

Patient: More when I'm doing something.

Doctor: Do you wake up at night not being able to breathe?

Patient: No, I don't think so.

Doctor: Are you wheezing or coughing?

Patient: Yes, some.

Doctor: Are you coughing up mucous?

Patient: Maybe a little.

Doctor: Do you have fever or chills?

Patient: Sometimes chills.

Doctor: Please sit on the exam table so that I can listen to your lungs.

DOLOR DE HOMBROS – SHOULDER PAIN

Doctor: ¿Puede indicar dónde le duele el hombro?

Patient: Aquí.

Doctor: ¿Se lastimó el hombro?

Patient: Sí, me caí sobre él.

Doctor: ¿Le duele llevar a cabo actividades diarias tales como peinarse?

Patient: Sí, me duele cuando lo muevo.

Doctor: ¿Siente entumecimiento, hormigueo o debilidad en el brazo?

Patient: Tengo el brazo muy débil.

Doctor: ¿Tiene el hombro hinchado?

Patient: Sí, creo que sí.

Doctor: ¿Siente a veces que el hombro se le sale de la cuenca?

Patient: No estoy segura.

Doctor: Le voy a revisar el arco de movimiento y fuerza muscular.

SHOULDER PAIN

Doctor: Can you point to where your shoulder hurts?

Patient: Right here.

Doctor: Did you injure your shoulder?

Patient: Yes, I fell on it.

Doctor: Is it painful to do any daily activities such as combing your hair?

Patient: Yes, it hurts whenever I move it.

Doctor: Do you have any numbness, tingling, or weakness in your arm?

Patient: My arm is very weak.

Doctor: Do you have any swelling in your shoulder?

Patient: Yes, I think so.

Doctor: Does your shoulder ever feel like it is coming out of its socket?

Patient: I'm not sure.

Doctor: I'm going to check your range of motion and your muscle strength.

DOLOR DE LA GARGANTA – SORE THROAT

Doctor: ¿Hace cuántos días que tiene dolor de garganta?

Patient: Tres días, doctor.

Doctor: ¿Está mejorando, empeorando, o sigue igual?

Patient: Más o menos igual.

Doctor: ¿Ha tenido faringitis alguna vez?

Patient: No lo creo.

Doctor: ¿Todavía tiene amígdalas?

Patient: No, doctor.

Doctor: Le voy a frotar dentro de la garganta.

Patient: Bueno.

Doctor: Abra bien la boca ...

SORE THROAT

Doctor: How many days have you had your sore throat?

Patient: Three days, doctor.

Doctor: Is it getting better, worse, or staying the same?

Patient: About the same.

Doctor: Have you ever had a strep infection?

Patient: I don't think so.

Doctor: Do you still have your tonsils?

Patient: No, doctor.

Doctor: I am going to swab your throat.

Patient: Okay.

Doctor: Open wide ...

INFECCIÓN RESPIRATORIA SUPERIOR – UPPER RESPIRATORY INFECTION

Doctor: ¿Cuánto tiempo hace que está enfermo?

Patient: Quizás tres días.

Doctor: ¿Tiene congestionados los senos nasales?

Patient: Sí.

Doctor: ¿Le sale mucosidad cuando se suena la nariz?

Patient: Sí.

Doctor: ¿Tiene infecciones de los senos frontales con frecuencia?

Patient: Sí, todos los inviernos.

Doctor: ¿Le han hecho cirugía de los senos frontales?

Patient: No.

Doctor: Le voy a dar golpecitos en las mejillas. Dígame si le duele.

Patient: Está bien.

UPPER RESPIRATORY INFECTION

Doctor: How long have you been sick?

Patient: Maybe three days.

Doctor: Do your sinuses feel congested?

Patient: Yes.

Doctor: Are you getting mucous when you blow your nose?

Patient: Yes.

Doctor: Do you get a lot of sinus infections?

Patient: Yes, every winter.

Doctor: Have you had sinus surgery?

Patient: No.

Doctor: I'm going to tap your cheeks. Tell me if it hurts.

Patient: Okay.

INFECCIÓN DEL APARATO URINARIO – URINARY TRACT INFECTION

Doctor: ¿Siente ardor al orinar?

Patient: Sí.

Doctor: ¿Orina con más frecuencia de lo usual?

Patient: Sí.

Doctor: Cuando tiene ganas, ¿siente que debe orinar inmediatamente?

Patient: Sí.

Doctor: Después de orinar, ¿siente que todavía le queda orina en la vejiga?

Patient: Sí, doctor.

Doctor: ¿Ha notado sangre en la orina?

Patient: No, no la he notado.

Doctor: Necesitamos una muestra de orina.

URINARY TRACT INFECTION

Doctor: Do you have a burning pain when you urinate?

Patient: Yes.

Doctor: Are you urinating more often than usual?

Patient: Yes.

Doctor: When you get the urge, do you feel that you must urinate immediately?

Patient: Yes.

Doctor: After urinating, does it feel like there is still urine in your bladder?

Patient: Yes, doctor.

Doctor: Have you noticed any blood in your urine?

Patient: No, I haven't noticed any.

Doctor: We need to take a urine sample ...

Conclusion

Thank you again for purchasing this book!

We hope this book was able to help you to improve your medical Spanish comprehension and vocabulary. Your new skillset speaking medical Spanish will help bring down language barriers and allow you to provide excellent care to those in need.

The next step is to continue putting your newly learned words and phrases to use in real world situations.

We congratulate you for completing this book and wish you all the best in your Spanish learning journey.

ABOUT THE AUTHOR

Touri is an innovative language education brand that is disrupting the way we learn languages. Touri has a mission to make sure language learning is not just easier but engaging and a ton of fun.

Besides the excellent books that they create, Touri also has an active website, which offers live fun and immersive 1-on-1 online language lessons with native instructors at nearly anytime of the day.

Additionally, Touri provides the best tips to improving your memory retention, confidence while speaking and fast track your progress on your journey to fluency.

Check out https://touri.co for more information.

OTHER BOOKS BY TOURI

GERMAN

Conversational German Dialogues: 50 German Conversations and Short Stories

German Short Stories (Volume 1): 10 Exciting Short Stories to Easily Learn German & Improve Your Vocabulary

ITALIAN

Conversational Italian Dialogues: 50 Italian Conversations and Short Stories

Italian Short Stories (Volume 1): 10 Exciting Short Stories to Easily Learn Italian & Improve Your Vocabulary

SPANISH

Conversational Spanish Dialogues: 50 Spanish Conversations and Short Stories

Spanish Short Stories (Volume 1): 10 Exciting Short Stories to Easily Learn Spanish & Improve Your Vocabulary

Spanish Short Stories (Volume 2): 10 Exciting Short Stories to Easily Learn Spanish & Improve Your Vocabulary

Intermediate Spanish Short Stories (Volume 1): 10 Amazing Short Tales to Learn Spanish & Quickly Grow Your Vocabulary the Fun Way!

Intermediate Spanish Short Stories (Volume 2): 10 Amazing Short Tales to Learn Spanish & Quickly Grow Your Vocabulary the Fun Way!

100 Days of Real World Spanish: Useful Words & Phrases for All Levels to Help You Become Fluent Faster

Learn Medical Spanish in 100 Days: Spanish Words & Phrases for Healthcare Professionals to Become Fluent Faster

FRENCH

Conversational French Dialogues: 50 French Conversations and Short Stories

French Short Stories for Beginners (Volume 1): 10 Exciting Short Stories to Easily Learn French & Improve Your Vocabulary

French Short Stories for Beginners (Volume 2): 10 Exciting Short Stories to Easily Learn French & Improve Your Vocabulary

Intermediate French Short Stories (Volume 1): 10 Amazing Short Tales to Learn French & Quickly Grow Your Vocabulary the Fun Way!

PORTUGUESE

Conversational Portuguese Dialogues: 50 Portuguese Conversations and Short Stories

ARABIC

Conversational Arabic Dialogues: 50 Arabic Conversations and Short Stories

RUSSIAN

Conversational Russian Dialogues: 50 Russian Conversations and Short Stories

CHINESE

Conversational Chinese Dialogues: 50 Chinese Conversations and Short Stories

ONE LAST THING...

If you enjoyed this book or found it useful, we would be very grateful if you posted a short review on Amazon.

Your support really does make a difference and we read all the reviews personally. Your feedback will make this book even better.

Thanks again for your support!

FREE SPANISH VIDEO COURSE

200+ words and phrases in audio

you can start using today!

Get it while it's available

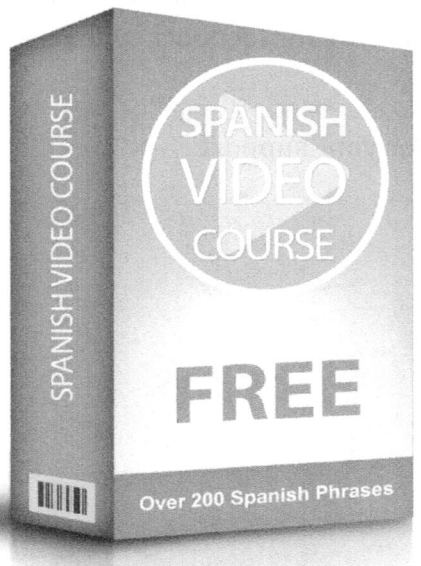

https://bit.ly/Medical-Spanish-Free-Video-Course

FREE AUDIOBOOKS

Touri has partnered with AudiobookRocket.com!

If you love audiobooks, here is your opportunity to get the NEWEST audiobooks completely FREE!

Thrillers, Fantasy, Young Adult, Kids, African-American Fiction, Women's Fiction, Sci-Fi, Comedy, Classics and many more genres!

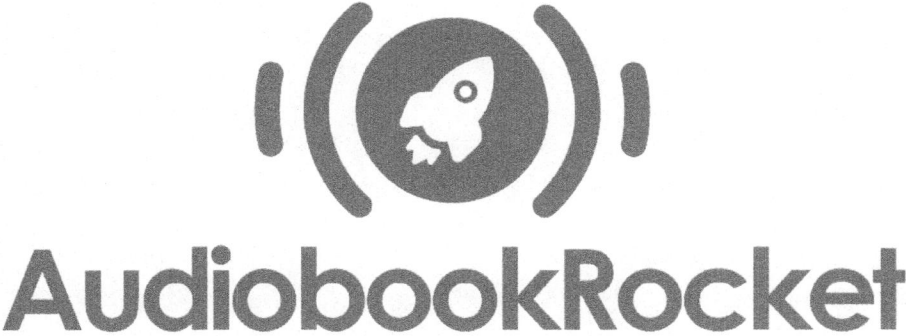

Visit AudiobookRocket.com!

Made in the USA
Monee, IL
07 July 2026

56546300R00164